Challenging The Dragon

FLYIN-BLIND

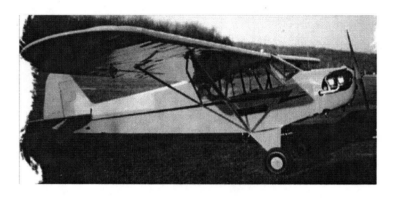

http://www.14ushop.com/flyin-blind
(Personal M.S. Web Site)
Living with a "Challenge"
and still being me.
Sequel to "M.S., My Story, Merciful Saviour"
First printing: Fall, 1998
Copyright © 2006 Jim Haverlock
ISBN: 1-4196-3181-0

To order additional copies, please contact us.
BookSurge, LLC
www.booksurge.com
1-866-308-6235
orders@booksurge.com

JIM HAVERLOCK

CHALLENGING THE DRAGON

2006

Challenging The Dragon

CONTENTS

DEFINITIONS
(For fun only)

PAIN:

"An uncomfortable frame of mind that may have a physical basis in something that is being done to the body, or may be purely mental, caused by the good fortune of another."

LIFE:

"A spiritual pickle preserving the body from decay."

"We live in daily apprehension of its loss; yet when lost it is not missed. The question, 'Is life worth living?' has been much discussed; particularly by those who think it is not, many of whom have written at great length in support of their view and by careful observance of the laws of health enjoyed for long terms of years the honors of successful controversy."

AGE:

"That period of life in which we compound for the vices that we still cherish by reviling those that we have no longer the enterprise to commit."

Definitions from "The Devil's Dictionary"

By Ambrose Bierce—compiled starting 1880

ACKNOWLEDGEMENTS

Cover picture credit goes to Emily Laguzza, age 14, daughter of Kristi Laguzza Boosman. I send a great big "thank you" to Emily for her gift of the original picture, and for her permission to use it for this cover.

I extend heartfelt thanks also to Glo Shemorry, a wonderful friend, who has written several books of her own, penned many songs, was a country-western singer, helped her husband, Bill, with his writing and photography and yet found time to write the "Holographic Imprints of a Man in Verse and Rhyme" which she consented to place in the pages of this book. Thank you, Glo, for your friendship and help.

And to Ron Foreman, I extend a bear hug for his friendship first, and for taking time to write the 'foreword' to this book. It is not widely known, but Ron is a direct descendant of Jane Seymour who was married for a short time to King Henry the VIII. One can truly say of Ron that he has blue blood running through his veins. Ron also traveled extensively and has lived in several countries after growing up in London, England. Thank you, Ron.

And a special "arigato goziamasu domo" to Dr. Anthony G. Payne, for his steadfast friendship and for putting up with all of my questions regarding stem cells, what ails me and all about living life to the fullest. Thank you also for taking time to review and edit this written expression of what is in my heart, and for graciously writing the Introduction. I could not have managed any of this without his advice and critique.

Thanks, too, to Pam Purtell, for truly putting up with me on a daily basis, eight hours a day in the confines of our internet-centered business office. Pam has three children, 2 boys and 1 girl and as you can imagine, she is as busy as a bee at all times.

And last but by no means least, joyous thanks to my family, for your prayers and expressions of concern, and for allowing me to live my life independently and as I see fit; for letting me be me.

The illustrations throughout this book are my own variations, to add another dimension.

Stem Cells

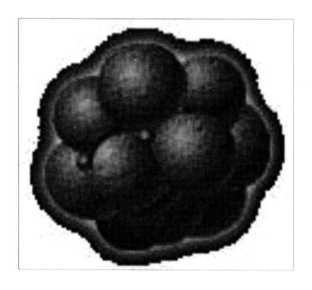

INTRODUCTION
By Dr. Anthony G. Payne

While teaching a class of university students in Japan during 2003, I drew upon the historic account of Gen. George Armstrong Custer's defeat on June 26, 1876 to illustrate an inescapable aspect of life:

"Friends, we are all headed to the *Little Big Horn.* Whether you get there as a young person or during middle-age or as a very old man or woman, ..we all have to the enter the valley and depart this world. No one escapes this fate. But as you correctly surmised, it isn't that final battle *alone* that determines the meaning and value of the life you have lived, but what you do in the days, weeks, and years leading up to it. And yes, the impact of your life and the ripples it sets in motion are determined by the choices and subsequent actions you take while en route to the valley."

http://14ushop.com/wizard/quick-bytes.htm#anchor3

Years later I would make the acquaintance of Jim Haverlock, a man who lives in the shadow of 2 valleys—one a literal valley (Methow Valley, Washington state) and the other a metaphorical one, but no less real (*The Valley of the Shadow of Death*). What he has managed to do and pull off while negotiating his way through the shadow lands of both is predicated on a rich blend of attitudes, practices and undertakings that are thought-provoking, awe-inspiring and heartwarming. His is a story that goes beyond one man's struggle with an insidious disease

(Multiple Sclerosis); indeed, in Jim's life story are found keen lessons and insights that apply to each of us, for surely we all wrestle with our own individual demons and dragons, as well as a host of issues related to our vulnerabilities and mortality. I cannot but believe there is something in the pages that follow for everyone.

"We who lived in concentration camps can remember the men who walked through the huts comforting others, giving away their last piece of bread. They may have been few in number, but they offer sufficient proof that everything can be taken from a man but one thing: the last of the human freedoms—to choose one's attitude in any given set of circumstances."

Victor Frankl, M.D.

FOREWARD
By Ronald Foreman

Once in a while, not often you understand but just once in a great while, it has been my privilege to meet and get to know an exceptional person really well. This does not happen often since most of us, and I include myself, tend to suppress or at least hide our interest in another person for fear of rejection or ridicule. Speaking as one of the vast majority I have little fear of contradiction when I say that neither rejection nor ridicule are particularly helpful in encouraging friendship. But then, as I said, once in a great while someone comes along who triggers the thought: 'I would really like to know that man' and caution goes with the wind.

It's been some years now since I met Jim Haverlock who at that time was establishing a foothold in the real estate business in Washington State. Those who have read Jim's book: 'M.S., My Story' will know of the events that preceded and followed the diagnosis of his illness as ALS (Lou Gehrig's Disease) and I will not attempt to discuss them here. It is sufficient to say that Jim took his many problems as a challenge that he needed to overcome and while he has had to acknowledge his illness he has never accepted it as incurable. From the beginning he felt that the three to five years given him by his physician was totally unacceptable and since at the time of this writing he is well into his Twelfth post diagnosis year—and heading for at least another twenty five—might be reasonable to assume that somebody had miscalculated. However, I prefer the alternative thought which is simply that Jim Haverlock can be an extremely resolute man who has decided to win this battle and he may well just do that.

Over the years he has developed a voluminous correspondence with fellow sufferers all over the world and many have marveled at his compassion and understanding, qualities that can only come in the world of MS when you can say: "Been there, done that."

Jim Haverlock is no saint, so very few of us are, but he is indeed an exceptional person who has never given me cause to regret my original thought: 'I would really like to know that man.' After all these years I am still working at it.

Ronald P. Foreman

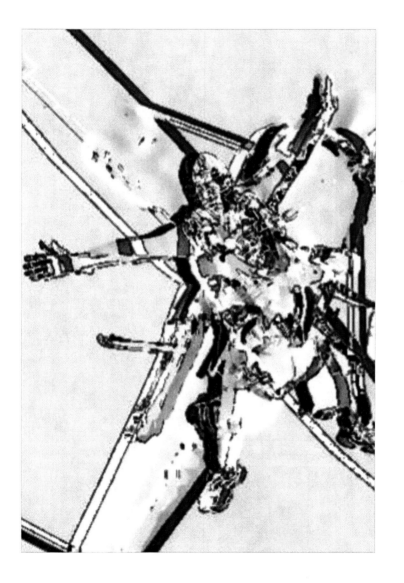

FREE FALL
A glimpse back...

Ohhhh! No turning back now!"

"We were face down with our arms and legs spread-eagled. The tandem master opened a small chute to slow our fall to about one-hundred twenty-five miles per hour. The wind rushed at us, making the skin on my face move while the jump suit flapped in the wind. I held my breath in the first few seconds of the fall then relaxed. As we passed through a thin cloud, the cameraman filming our descent appeared in front of me and just a few feet below. There was sixty exhilarating seconds of free-fall before the chute opened. I felt the jolt as we went from flat fall to upright and slowed abruptly to thirty-five miles per hour."

"My life, after all, has been a free fall. God had provided me with a joyful way to experience my faith. I was wholly willing to let go knowing I had a Merciful Savior. Then I did let go. It was fantastic!

Simply *f a n t a s t i c*!

It has been more than 6 years since those words were written as the ending of my first book, a book that opened up my life to the world. As scary as it was back then (and still is) to share one's "diary of life", I can honestly look back today and say: "It was worth every minute of the effort, resources and opening of this soul—to all those who would read the words expressed."

Why? You may ask. And the answer:

Doors and hearts have opened, new friendships have been made, words of encouragement have been offered, prayers by fellow spirits fill the unbounded plane, things thought impossible have proven 'possible', and life continues to be rich, full and exciting; a journey whose path has afforded unending possibilities, joys and rewards, as well as trials, tribulations and sorrows. Living life one day at a time, like we all should do, and the great 'sages' admonished, makes this earthly journey a most joyous experience.

My life is much like an artist's canvas bearing images, colors and hues that are a heady mix of vibrant and dark; a wondrous painting dotted with all the ups and downs that make this enterprise we call life worth having lived. I speak of seeing children grow into wonderful people with children of their own; meeting fellow travelers who walk similar paths to mine; witnessing the sun rise anew each day, and the sunsets that welcome the night; experiencing the joys and sorrows of family and friends;

Sorrows such as—loss of close friends as their season ends; shedding tears of compassion for those grieving their loss; shouldering the failures and hurts that family and friends go through; and dwelling at times in that valley which is filled with the daily tribulations we all witness and live. For in reality, life is all this and more, a mix of good and bad, joyous and sorrowful, burdens and carefree moments, love and it's loss, and certainly the occasional touch of mourning or grieving.

Experiencing life daily with an added "challenge" such as Multiple Sclerosis can be rewarding, although not without difficulties and the feeling of "loss" as what is 'normal' and taken for granted is compromised or lost. All those living with MS, or any other debilitating "challenge", go through a continual 'grieving' process. 'Grieving' over each bodily faculty which does not work as well as it use to—or not at all. It is a process that casts long shadows over each day and sometimes threatens to eclipse the sun.

How is this in any way, shape or form "Rewarding"?

It is...

And how so you ask?

Take my hand and join me now on this journey in the pages that follow, and discover thereby the possibilities that announce themselves to us all on a daily basis. Witness life through the eyes of one seeking a 'healing', a 'miracle', while learning what life truly is about; a quest for the meaning of life that for this writer includes the motive for hammering out this tome: Helping but not judging others, and loving all of creation. For as my friend, Dr. Anthony G. Payne so aptly expressed—"Our material possessions and honors are left at the foot of the grave. The only thing we take beyond the doors of 'Forest Lawn' is our deeds."

CHAPTER I
What About Dragons?

Over the years I have come to totally detest using the label given by doctors for my condition, namely M.S. I have chosen not to allow my mind and brain to get so absorbed with what those initials stand for by today's reckoning. Instead I have chosen to call this "my challenge", for indeed it is just that, a real life challenge. And by this I mean:

A challenge to overcome each loss of function as it occurs; a challenge to maintain one's identity as a real human being and not be ostracized as the lepers and sick people mentioned within the Bible of old were; a challenge to keep smiling in spite of setbacks and complications; a challenge to surmount in terms of creating a viable money-making business; a challenge in the sense that it continually brings me back to who I really am and what really matters most in this journey from cradle to grave.

It is a challenge much like what folks associate with "dragons". After all, dragons are portrayed as evil, vicious, man-eating monsters. It is an image that inspired the title of this book—Challenging the Dragon. And it is an image that bears fleshing out.

Consider the dragons from the Western Tradition:

Western dragons aren't necessarily evil—but they often are. At the very least they tend to be solitary and bad-tempered.

The typical Western dragon—or Wyrm—is a large, scaly creature resembling a dinosaur or a large lizard. It usually has wings and can fly, often it will breathe fire.

Western dragons tend to live in caves in mountains or hidden away in the forests. They often guard a stash of gold. Western dragons are often used to symbolize greed.

Dragons vary as much as people do. Although many Western dragons are brutal, ignorant creatures that kill and eat humans—others are portrayed as wise creatures more akin to those found in the Far East.

Western dragons are seen as being distinctly different from their Eastern counterparts. Legends originating in European countries portray dragons as giant winged fire-breathing creatures that are usually feared by humans.

Many stories tell of men who battle against all obstacles to fight the scary dragons, get past them and gain access to the riches and wealth hidden in dragon dens. The epic hero, Beowulf, is just one example of someone who attempted to fight a treasure-guarding dragon—although in his case he failed and was killed.

The defining characteristic of a Western dragon symbol is that it represents power. Having an image of a Western dragon can help in expressing feelings of self-esteem, but they're also popular with dragon fans.

Now let's consider the Eastern Dragon Tradition:

The symbol of the dragon represents a spiraling day.

The Celestial Chinese Dragon is comparable as the symbol of the Chinese race itself. Chinese around the world, proudly proclaim themselves "Lung Tik Chuan Ren" (Descendents of the Dragon). Dragons are referred to as the divine mythical creature that brings with it ultimate abundance, prosperity and good fortune.

As the emblem of the Emperor and the Imperial order, the legend of the Chinese Dragon permeates ancient Chinese civilization and shaped the evolution of their culture. Its benevolence signifies greatness, goodness and blessings.

The Chinese Dragon, or Lung , symbolizes power and excellence, valiancy and boldness, heroism and perseverance, nobility and divinity. A dragon overcomes obstacles until success is his. He is energetic, decisive, optimistic, intelligent and ambitious.

Unlike the negative energies associated with Western Dragons, most Eastern Dragons are beautiful, friendly, and wise. They are the angels of the Orient. Instead of being hated, they are loved and worshipped. Temples and shrines have been built to honor them, for they control the rain, rivers, lakes, and seas. Many Chinese cities have pagodas where people used to burn incense and pray to dragons. The Black Dragon Pool Chapel, near Peking, was reserved for the Empress and her court.

The 4 Dragons: A Chinese Tale

Once upon a time, there were no rivers and lakes on earth, but only the Eastern Sea, in which lived four dragons: the Long Dragon, the Yellow Dragon, the Black Dragon and the Pearl Dragon.

One day the four dragons flew from the sea into the sky. They soared and dived, playing at hide-and-seek in the clouds.

"Come over here quickly!" the Pearl Dragon cried out suddenly.

"What's up?" asked the other three, looking down in the direction where the Pearl Dragon pointed. On the earth they saw many people putting out fruits and cakes, and burning incense sticks. They were praying! A white-haired woman, kneeling on the ground with a thin boy on her back, murmured:

"Please send rain quickly, God of Heaven, to give our children rice to eat.."

There had been no rain for a very long time and as a result the crops had withered, the grass had turned yellow and the fields cracked under the scorching sun.

"How poor the people are!" said the Yellow Dragon. "And they will die if it doesn't rain soon."

The Long Dragon nodded. Then he suggested, "Let's go and beg the Jade Emperor for rain."

So saying, he leapt into the clouds. The others followed closely and flew towards the Heavenly Palace.

Being in charge of all the affairs in heaven, on earth and in the sea, the Jade Emperor was very powerful. He was not pleased to see the dragons rushing in. "Why do you come here instead of staying in the sea and behaving yourselves?"

The Long Dragon stepped forward and said, "The crops on earth are withering and dying, Your Majesty. I beg you to send rain down quickly!"

"Alright, you go back first and I'll send some rain down tomorrow." The Jade Emperor pretended to agree while listening to the songs of fairies hovering nearby.

"Thanks, Your Majesty!" And with this the four dragons returned home.

But ten days passed, and not a drop of rain came down.

The people suffered more, some (in fact) began eating bark, some grass roots. And when this was exhausted, the ravenous souls began eating white clay.

Seeing all this, the four dragons felt very sorry, for they knew the Jade Emperor only cared about pleasure, and never took the people's plight to heart. They could only rely on themselves to relieve the people of their miseries. But how to do it?

Seeing the vast sea, the Long Dragon said that he had an idea.

"What is it? Out with it, quickly!" the other three demanded.

"Look, is there not plenty of water in the sea where we live? We should scoop it up and spray it towards the sky. The water will be like rain drops and come down to save the people and their crops."

"Good idea!" The others clapped their hands.

"But," said the Long Dragon after thinking a bit, "we will incur the Jade Emperor's wrath if he ever learns of this."

"I will do anything to save the people," the Yellow Dragon said resolutely.

"Let's begin. We will never regret it." The Black Dragon and the Pearl Dragon were not to be outdone.

They flew to the sea, scooped up water in their mouths, and then flew back into the sky, where they sprayed the water out over the earth. The four dragons flew back and forth, making the sky dark all around. Before long the seawater became rain pouring down from the sky.

"It's raining! It's raining!"

"The crops will be saved!"

The people cried and leaped with joy. On the ground the wheat stalks raised their heads and the sorghum stalks straightened up.

The god of the sea discovered these events and reported it to the Jade Emperor.

"How dare the four dragons bring rain without my permission!" The Jade Emperor shouted. Enraged now, he ordered his heavenly generals and their troops to arrest the four dragons. Being far outnumbered, the four dragons could not defend themselves, and they were soon arrested and brought back to the heavenly palace.

"Go and get four mountains to lie upon them so that they can never escape!" The Jade Emperor commanded of the Mountain God.

The Mountain God used his magic power to make four mountains uproot, fly to where the dragons were, and press down upon them.

Imprisoned as they were, the dragons never regretted their actions. Determined to do good for the people always, they turned themselves into four rivers, which flowed past high mountains and deep valleys, crossing the land from the west to the east and finally emptying into the sea. And so China's four great rivers were formed—the Heilongjian (Black Dragon) in the far north, the Huanghe (Yellow River) in central China, the Changjiang (Yangtze, or Long River) farther south, and the Zhujiang (Pearl) in the very far south.

CHAPTER TWO
"Seek and ye shall find"

This is a familiar saying most of us have heard in our lifetime, at least in a passing sort of way. Seriously taken by many, forgotten by others, it has been broadcast world wide for at least a couple of thousand years.

What do these words have to do with any life and/or especially for a life with a neurological & immune challenge?

The first time I heard this phrase was at a very early age, spoken by a Benedictine Catholic nun, a catechism teacher. At the age of six they did not have much meaning, if any at all, and went unheeded, lying dormant, as most seeds do, until watered, nurtured and cultivated by caring hands.

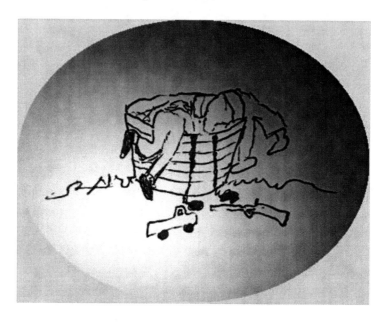

Oil Painting ©

When only three, my friend and me
Were left in the care
Of our dads who were there
Busily working and visiting, too,
While ma was at church doing what
Church women do, when we
Spotted a tub full of old
Crank-case oil, and smack in
The middle, a mysterious foil
That looked like a bird that was
Draped all in black, a pitiful
Sight, like a blown out old sack,
Then grabbing a stick to poke and

To prod, we lifted it out cuz we
Knew that God would not want
To leave it in there for to die,
So we rescued the thing and
Breathed a big sigh; were we
Ever surprised when we found
That our bag was nothing indeed
But a dirty old rag; of course
We dripped oil from our ribs by
This time but decided we'd head
For the kitchen and prime
Ourselves with some cookies
And kool aid as we had just
Finished a project as big
As could be, our hands slid
On walls and cupboards and
Doors, but the look on ma's
Face really gave us the
Horrors, she grabbed a chair,
guess she thought she
was fainting, from
viewing my first and only
oil painting.

As the years sped by and I made my way through grade
school, these words still lie dormant, or so I thought. In reality
though, I was subconsciously seeking—body and mind. At
first my seeking was confined to "fun things," as children are
drawn to, such as the cookies my mother had carefully hidden
away from my sister, brother and me; then came seeking the
approval of others for my accomplishments. This early seeking

was followed by mastery of the A, B, C's, reading, arithmetic, geography, history, and religion.

Looking for or seeking things—be it knowledge or opportunities or what-have-you—is a characteristic most of us readily identify with our forefathers and also with those of us who happen to grow up in "rustic settings". I grew up in North Dakota in a family that was about as rustic or frontier-*sy* as one could get. My father built our 4 room house as well as an attached four car garage and repair shop he owned and ran. By age six I was stoking our stove with coal hauled in from a mill six miles down the road, and also swept the floors and washed machine parts in gasoline for my father. I was always greasy, oiling and reeking of gas. By the time I was ten I could take out a Chevy motor and completely strip it in one hour flat.

Home ©

Dad built it himself
With the skills he had grown
To depend on and so he designed
Our first home out of old railroad ties
That he'd scavenged and saved,
A castle indeed for ma
Who just raved that she had three rooms,
The kids room and theirs' off limits to us
Even for prayers
The rest of the house was just one room
But then we ate in its kitchen'
Which turned into a den
Of everyone living in everyone's sight
With even a phone that rang day and night
A party line ringing out good news and bad,

Bringing in jobs for my busy dad
So he added a garage with four stalls
Thru the wall ma would holler to him
When he'd get a call
Then she'd push back her hair
From her face and she'd run
To buy parts for my dad
So's to get the job done
In a car that purred softly
Because Dad was the best
A repair man whose work stood up to the test
Often she'd leave her scrub board
To go, a respite indeed
(for those who don't know)
from scrubbing our clothes
and wringing by hand
she'd just leave them soak
do what life would demand
grandpa would drop off chickens to eat
our bellies were filled by their juices so sweet
the grocery store just a couple blocks down
our school to the north
farm land all around
with a tavern and pool hall
a church that stood tall
south of our house
reminding us all
to count our blessings
although I should add
two elevators stood in good years or bad
yawning for harvest
for then farmers could

pay as dad favored them
often in his generous way
railroad tracks lay a block
from our door for a boy
who liked dreaming
you'd not ask for more
still each time I'd listen
to that whistle blow
my mind stole to places
I longed to go

By the time I reached the final year of grade school I had
managed to accumulate enough money to buy a 1929 Model
A Ford—forty dollars! I then set about cleaning and repairing
it—then painted it black and red on the outside with a yellow
interior. It wasn't long after that that folks would routinely
spot me driving down local streets.

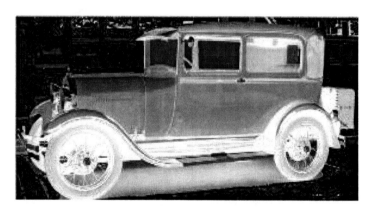

My First Car ©

The junker I'd found
And for it I paid
Just forty dollars
From money I'd saved
Then I painted and
Prodded, hammered and
Hummed, til that junker
Became a magnificent one.
I painted it's chassis
A bright red and yellow
It purred like a kitten,
What you'd expect
From a fellow
With taste so sublime
Who'd taken the time
To cover the cushions
With a leopard design.
With the power of a mule
Always ready to go; it
Succumbed to my moods
Whether fast or slow.
Some laughed,
"a monstrosity's'
decided to roam", but
those days that I
drove the nuns
to their home
the town folk would turn
give a wave of their hand
as though I were driving
a queens mini van.
I was only thirteen

But with skills
I had learned
In my father's garage,
My heart and hands
Turned some junk
Into motion; I was
Proud I could say
It was mine cuz I'd
Earned that old Model A.

I graduated eighth grade as class valedictorian and set my sights on becoming a priest. There was a local religious high school, but I had my heart set on leaving home and attending high school at Crosier Seminary in Onamia, Minnesota. It took some finagling, but this is exactly where I landed—in the midst of a school that played host to some two hundred and fifty students and forty priests and monks (brothers)—and a farm.

During my first summer break, I went home and proudly announced that I would not be working in Dad's shop, but instead would find my own job. And I did, working for a local farmer who'd agreed to pay me $8 day plus room and board. After working from dawn to dusk for two straight weeks, I was paid the grand sum of $10. It turned out the farmer couldn't afford any more than this. I had been double-crossed and, well, this bit of opportunity seeking had not turned out so well.

Not being one to sit on my business end, I got busy and landed a job working for a beekeeper. This time I got paid what was due me, but there was a big bonus: The apiary owner taught me to fly his little J3 cub airplane. And fly I did—taking the plane all over the place and doing things in it that my father called the acts of a "crazy daredevil."

Following my graduation from high school in 1957, I enrolled in Dickinson State University and began studying business and accounting. In my spare time I continued my work at the apiary, which earned me enough money to pay for my tuition, books, clothes, and room and board. I also began to socialize more and found myself at a local dance partnered up with a girl named Gorgianne. Now priests-in-the-making certainly have been known to date before taking their vows, so there was nothing untoward about my taking to the dance floor with a pretty girl. But there was something untoward about how frisky this gal made me feel and, in the weeks and months to come I knew that hormones were winning out over my best intentions. Not wanting to "wallow in sin", I asked Gorgianne to marry me and over my family's protests, we were wed in December 1958.

School ©

Between our house and the
River, our village school
Stood, a monument credit
Built by those who could
Dream that with knowledge,
Persistence and might, and
God's help to guide us,
We could better our plight.
It's brown brick was in
Contrast to the grass
'neath its hill, snow in
winter provided us all
with a thrill as we slid
down its surface

again and again, with no
thought of the future, or
homework, or sin; it's bell
tolled the tidings that
school had begun, and it
clanged a reminder
when classwork was done.
The skirts of the Sisters
Would swish in a way,
Warning God listened
To each word we would say,
So we'd best be chaste,
Stay virgin and humble or
The heavens would turn and
Create quite a rumble. One
Room I avoided as much
As I could, was where books
All went begging because
I never would
Pick up one more profound
Than the National Geo; though
On the gym floor, I was a
Regular Leo; Though shy in the
Classroom, I never did fail,
But shamed by the Sister,
From her slap and her rail;
I dreamed of her torture
By Indians who'd stake
With wet ties of leather
In the sun she would bake
And after the vultures
Had transposed her remains

Her bones would still shiver
From late summer rains.
But there was another
So gentle and kind
I hold in dreams still
Etched in my mind
For no greater lesson
In school did I learn
Than the sweetness of life
When love is returned;
The day of her transfer
I felt heaven's first tug
When she leaned over to give me
My very first hug.

I continued working for the apiary, but in time landed a position as an accountant for Conlin Furniture and spent the next nine years doing my "bookkeeping thing". When the manager got ill with cancer and eventually died, I was made manager and soon found myself working longer hours than ever before. During this time I took the measly $500 I had managed to save up during my tenure with Conlin, and used it as a down payment on two rental houses. Less than two years later I borrowed the money to buy an eight unit apartment building. I now was clearing some good money and even had enough surplus capital to return to flying, which I had not done in over thirteen years!

In 1972 the owner of Conlin Furniture, Clem Conlin, and I formed a partnership and opened Budget Furniture, and hired a manager to run it for us. I oversaw things there, but continued to manage Conlin Furniture. Things were moving and growing, as was my family—eight children!

Seekers keep seeking.

During July 1973 I ran across two North Dakota furniture stores for sale, one in Devil's Lake and the other in Carrington, and wound up buying both. Intent on leaving Conlin Furniture now, I tried to resign—but was persuaded by Clem Conlin to stay on. So for the next few years I was pretty much running four furniture stores!

My successes mounted, yes, but during all this my wife, Gorgianne and I had begun battling one another and drifted apart. Although I was trying hard to follow Catholic teachings and not divorce, this was the ultimate outcome. When the smoke cleared, my wife wound up being handed everything we'd accumulated—house, new car, cabin, boat and more.

I remained single for a few years, than plunged into a whirlwind romance, got married again, only to find that the new Mrs. Haverlock was chasing other men before the ink was dry on our marriage license. A 2nd divorce followed suit, naturally. As if this was not trouble enough, my partner Clem died as did the oil boom that sustained our region. As a result, my business declined while my debt went up—and after 4 years or so of battling having to close up shop, I finally called it a day.

Surely the time had come to seek out greener pastures— *anywhere*. Of course, starting over from scratch at forty-eight during a recession was daunting. Here I was, a guy who'd flown airplanes and owned and run many highly successful businesses, and I didn't seem to have any Chutzpah left. What I did have was fear and uncertainty. Thankfully I managed to get back on my feet over time—mainly by setting up accounts for furniture distributors. In time, my territory grew to include North & South Dakota, Montana, and the Carolinas—and I was made regional manager.

During this particular time my sister moved to North Carolina, followed by my parents. I had an apartment in South Carolina, which made visiting with immediate family a "hop, skip and a jump" affair.

I also branched out socially, having met a divorcee named Nell who had two teenage children living with her. We hit it off well and within a short span of time went from dating and long phone calls, to getting married. Since we were all smitten with South Carolinian beaches, we decided to make our home in Surfside Beach.

But within fifteen months the old ghosts of economic peril were to dog my steps: My employer (Soil Pruf) was facing economic problems and had to lay off many salesmen. My job was safe, but my salary had to be cut fifty percent. It wasn't long before I parted company with Soil Pruf to take on being manager of a small furniture store some thirty miles away from my home.

Two things emerged early on in the course of my new job: I began to notice that my legs didn't hold up so well when it came to hauling furniture to and fro. And secondly, I found that no amount of work or sacrifice pleased the owner, and as a result wound up resigning.

Seekers take calculated risks to get ahead, and I certainly had taken my fair share. In a way, we are like nomads traveling across a mighty desert, sometimes finding an oasis—and other times a dry hole. Of course, we can't always count on help or guidance from family, much less friends as we cross life's deserts—but by-and-large we do count on our bodies holding up and not letting us down. In fact we tend to take our mortal shell for granted, and even grow oblivious to its marvelous workings; that is, unless it begins to sputter and falter. This is what happened to me—on the heels of my "leg problems" at my last place of employment. Something was going wrong and it became impossible to ignore—especially following some physical tumbles I took while jogging. This set me to consciously seeking in earnest and with actual planning and foresight. Was I at age 54 too old for jogging? Is the body telling me to slow down? Is daily jogging not part of life when one gets older? How do I gain back control of my life? Why, why, why?

The first and most logical "next step" following my spate of stumbling was to have someone watch as I jogged. I wanted an observer to tell me if there was some physical reason for this tripping. When none could be seen (finding), I was quick to dismiss the problem as something that 'just happened' and would not likely occur ever again.

As the pavement and my body met brutally while walking from my car to a local post office some weeks later, the 'seeking' resumed albeit more earnestly. As the sores from this fall became scars, which slowly disappeared, the earnest quest for answers slowed also. At least until the next "trip" to the concrete took place! (Ouch!)

This state-of-affairs changed rather quickly and dramatically following an incident in which I took yet another fall, this time at a client's desk following a meeting. As if to add insult to injury, I became nauseated and experienced a severe headache that lasted the entire day. The time for ignoring the signals from my body was over, as was any pretense of seeking answers.

My first stop was a general practitioner MD, followed by a visit with a neurologist. I held out hope that he could explain what was happening, and more importantly why and how to fix whatever was mucking up my bodily works.

After eight months and more tests than I care to remember

or ever want to go through ever again, the diagnosis came down: I had an incurable, irreversible, swiftly debilitating neurological disorder—ALS. The disease that took famed baseball player Lou Gehrig's life and for which this disease was named ("Lou Gehrig's Disease"). Oddly, the diagnosis came on the heels of a lengthy visit to the Mayo Clinic—that wound up just before Thanksgiving!

It looked as though my life would soon be over. What should a man facing his own mortality do? Why, turn to his loved ones for comfort, of course. So I reached out to my wife—and received a rebuke. "It's over Jim, I'm not happy with you. I don't love you anymore. It's over". Surely, I thought, I was the turkey being carved up—heart first.

Now I really was on a quest; a quest to place all my troubles aside save one—ALS. I had to find out what this label meant, and what could be done to "deactivate" this insidious disease. I found out rather quickly that the treatments for my condition did little, except help one deal with specific symptoms. This realization gave rise in quick succession to disbelief, frustration, anger and finally some sense of surrender to what was transpiring.

After a couple of months of wallowing in self pity, complicated by the flight of my 'life partner' and the subsequent loss of my financial base, I was at my wits end. I wanted to surrender; to just wave a white flag and give up. But surrender to whom? I looked around—and then up. Yes, of course,...who else could possibly help a guy in my scuffed toed shoes...but the Almighty. I signed the "unconditional surrender papers" right then and there, offering up my body and life to a greater and higher power.

The surrender to a "higher power", to God, gave me peace of mind. Which is to say, peace from what had been constant concerns over having no financial means, as well as the 'how' of making a living, especially since no one would consider hiring a "disabled" person who would continue to worsen (Especially when there were so many younger, healthier people looking for work).

The total peace of mind that came with that act of complete surrender gave rise to a corresponding positive attitude. I somehow "knew that I knew that I knew" that this neurologic demon would not hold me in its grasp forever, but was something I would have to wrestle with in order to get better. This peace, I might add, was the greatest gift one could ever ask, hope or pray for.

PEACE, FAITH, LOVE, HOPE

Peace is something we all seek and desire, but at times it seems unattainable, so it leaves us.

Faith—as a child it seems so natural—faith that we will be cared for and loved—only to find out things are not so cozy in the real world. Sometimes this causes faith to wither and even die.

Love is the key, but during our days on this ancient space rock we see it wasted or used by many for greedy, selfish ends. And so love dies.

Hope—what good is hope?

The flame of Hope should never go out in our life....

For with HOPE each of us can live a life with......

PEACE, FAITH and LOVE

Even as this body continued 'tripping' and meeting the concrete, nose to cement mixed with sand and stone, the knowing that it would not last forever continued to fuel a positive attitude and thus inspire my daily life. This is not to say

I did not get angry, even mad at God who for whatever reason allowed this to happen, or that I escaped being depressed—for these certainly did occur. They just didn't hang around long. Most important was the peace and positive-ness which was becoming a way of living—and which came to dominate my life. I even found a saying that reflected my emerging mindset— one that was fun and captured my feelings succinctly: "I don't mind falling, I just hate hitting the ground!"

Seeking adventures while saddled with a physical challenge seemed almost natural back then, and continues to be a layer in my everyday life. The adventures have and do brighten my days and provide continued challenges and much enjoyment as was the case prior to my diagnosis, albeit differently. In retrospect, I came to see that many of the people who figured in these adventures predated my initial diagnosis and was almost strategically in-place when the proverbial diagnostic axe fell.

One of these early adventures occurred on the heels of a phone call that came my way one quiet day while I was sitting at home looking through area help wanted ads, seeking some form of employment. The male caller identified himself as "St. Clair" and, after getting acquainted, he proceeded to ask me to take a ride with him to a city some 60 miles away. Since I had no immediate or pressing plans, I quickly agreed as it would afford me the chance to hang out with a friendly soul and get out of the house in the bargain.

When we got to St. Clair's intended destination, I was led to a meeting with a man named Clark Greene and his wife. It didn't take long for the conversation to shift to Clark's history and (with this) the reason for the trip itself. It turned out that Clark also had MS and had taken a leap of faith and traveled to another country for treatment to aid his 'disability';

a treatment that had worked. Now he wanted to share his story and help someone else.

As his story unfolded as told by both Clark and his Mrs., I learned that they had children and that he, like me, had lost his job. Clark also talked at length about how his relationship with his wife and children had suffered in the wake of his condition. He then shared with me how he'd left home to see Dr. Hans Nieper in Germany, all the while bedeviled with constant severe headaches and pain. Now mind you, he could get about.....walking a distance of 3 city blocks in the 'quick time' of forty five minutes. After 2 weeks at Dr. Nieper's clinic, he returned home able to negotiate the stairs from the airplane with out any canes, and then swiftly walk up to his waiting family. Following his reunion, he went on to not only get his job back at a local steel mill, but to work full time to boot. And he began walking.... two miles each and every day. To say his life did a turnaround is an understatement!

This was great news, of course. Clark then handed me the fax number for Dr. Nieper's clinic and asked that I write up a one page summary of my condition and diagnosis and transmit it quickly. The clinic was often booked up, so all we could collectively hope for was that I would get an appointment a few months down the road.

Once I got back home my resolve to dash off a letter began to waver, mainly because there were no funds available to make this trip. I finally resolved to write and send it anyway, if only because I figured it would take months to get in to see Nieper; time enough to figure out how to come up with sufficient money to make the trip and pay for any exams or treatments he might prescribe.

The fax went out late sometime on a mid January evening. The next morning I was awaken by the ringing of my phone.

Being half awake, I stumbled over to the fax machine where a paper was now coming through. It was coming from the clinic in Germany and stated that an appointment had been made for two weeks hence, in early February. Apparently I was the beneficiary of a timeslot that opened up due to a cancellation.

Now what was I supposed to do? This wasn't supposed to happen so quickly! And where exactly was the money going to come from?

The only thing that came to mind was to call up my newfound friend, St. Clair and his friend, Clark and ask their advice. During the conversation that ensued, I mentioned that I would really have to cancel this appointment due to a lack of funds. Their reply was, 'keep the appointment, the money will be there'. With this reassurance came great inner calm, though I had to wonder how this was supposed to come about.

I then scrambled around and scraped together every free cent I could find, which wound up being about half of what I needed. Where was the other half going to come from? I had no other resources, no credit line for such a venture, and was convinced that no medical insurance would pay for services outside of the United States. Understanding little of how the Universe worked its subtle magic when allowed to do so, I continued to fret.

During the next weeks I paid for my air travel using the available funds. Dr. Nieper's clinic staff proceeded to make reservations for a room within walking distance of the clinic. A good-hearted friend who had family working for a major airline got a pass so he could travel along with me so as to be available to provide any assistance I might need. And unbeknownst to me, St. Clair quietly went about raising funds as did a former employer and his wife, along with other friends.

With only a few days left before my flight, these good

friends prepared a surprise dinner for me which saw some 70 people show up. Following our meal, the "ring leaders" sprang their big surprise on me—an envelope containing the other half of the funds I needed. Needless to say, I shed more than a few tears of joy—and relief.

In this instance, 'Seek and ye shall find' became more than just a matter of my seeking something, it became a group effort. For me, this was a valuable lesson learned late in a life concerning the limits of so-called 'independence', as well as the foolhardiness of being stubbornly self-sufficient, full of pride and ego. It was also a needed lesson in learning how to receive, as I had previously been the giver, expecting nothing in return. Then, too, though it was quite a challenge allowing others' to feel good about helping me, this too was something I needed to experience.

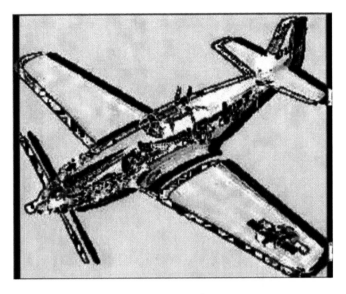

My Hero ©

With my trusty umbrella I'd parachute down
From the top of the roof in view of the town
Just hoping that someone somewhere would see
That no one was quite as courageous as me.
Then one day, much to my wondrous surprise,
I saw flying over with my pilot eyes a World
War II pilot buzzing over our town, I later
Found out he was looking around for his wife
Who was working just so she would know, he
Circled again just to wave her hello.
It was then I decided that one day I'd be a
Regular pilot and fly just like he; those
Throbbing engines, I felt to my toes; his face I
Saw clearly; now everyone knows that he was

JIM HAVERLOCK

My hero and others as well, though he never
Came home from that war of hell.

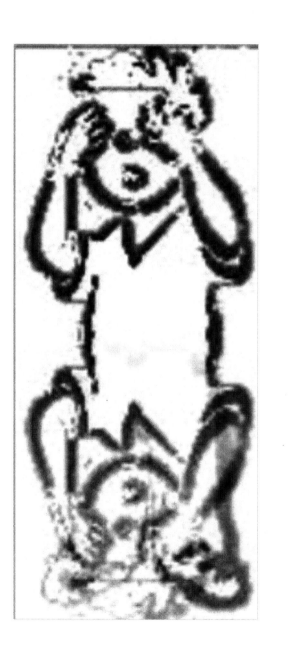

CHAPTER THREE
Hide and Seek

During my stay in Germany, Dr. Nieper did an exhaustive array of tests on me—and came up with a different diagnosis than my back home experts: He was absolutely sure that I had progressive MS and not ALS. This was a diagnosis I could live with—*literally*. I clung to the new diagnosis, and looked forward to his treatments with newfound hope and joy.

In the weeks to come I was given various treatments, the most effective being IVs of calcium ethanolamine phosphate (EAP) which helped my demyelinated nerves conduct electrical current better. Buoyed up by the German therapies, I returned to the States without the use of my canes and promptly fell into old, familiar "go it alone" patterns and habits. Of course, I had to think about making a living. And though I was better now, the fact remained I still had difficulties that would make prospective employers reluctant to take me on. With this in mind, I set about planning a new business venture. Having worked with furniture for many years, it was natural to look at that aspect and how it might fare in the area of South Carolina I lived in.

My little seaside community niche boasted many tourist attractions, namely the Atlantic Ocean, glitzy novelty stores, restaurants with low paying wages, numerous hotels and motels for guests to stay, apartments, condos, town houses and rental homes. It was also plagued by the defections of scores of locals who were moving to warmer parts of the country. After ruminating on all this for a while, I decided that a furnishings venture would be my best shot at creating a viable revenue generating machine.

In quick order thought turned to planning, then action. The feeling of being creative and productive again made me feel good, and it wasn't long before my grim countenance was replaced by a decidedly more cheery one. Much was missing, however.

During this time, I sold classified and little block ads which helped provide enough funds for a meager existence. While negotiating a new contact with a business owner, he mentioned how taking a retreat was great for helping one quietly "screw the head and mind back on so it would fit properly once again."

Within a few short days, this chap called and enthusiastically announced that he had a retreat site picked out: The Methow Valley of Washington State (North Cascade Mountains); specifically, our choice of a mountainside Teepee or house located in a little village bearing the quaint name of "Twisp". And, best of all, we wouldn't have to come up with a red cent for the retreat site, only for getting there.

Having never heard of the Methow Valley or Twisp (Native American Name for 'Hornets'), or of anyone offering a 'free' (no strings attached) anything, I was a bit incredulous. The business person who'd arranged all this picked up on my skepticism, placed a phone call, and handed me the phone. The voice on the other end was a man and his first words were—"Is this Jim?" "Are you on your way yet?"

I was taken aback, so much so that it was all I could do to remain calm let alone respond. The voice interjected: "It's

Brother Harry. Get yourself together and get on out here now, you have a choice of living in the house with me, or staying in a teepee on the side of a mountain in the countryside, alone. Make the choice when you get here. And, when will you be here anyway?"

I began to wonder just how much I really wanted to "duck out" of the mainstream and sit in a Teepee or house up on the side of a mountain on the opposite side of the country! However, I knew deep down that a retreat would provide a quiet place for just God and this 'disabled' person to get better acquainted and for me to 'seek' answers to perplexing, persistent questions.

It took only minutes for me to toss my doubts to the wind and leap with both feet into this new adventure. The die was now cast.

With the aid of a daughter who worked for one of the airlines, a parent pass was granted to me that allowed stopovers long enough for me to visit with family on the way to and from Seattle. My former worry was gone now, replaced instead by a sense of expectancy at seeing home folks and, more importantly, being with the Almighty and nature. Perhaps now I could sort my life out and come up with a firm sense of what direction to move in.

Even before my excursion to the Pacific Northwest began unexpected things cropped up that seem to help consolidate my course. Strangers offered advice or, conversely, sought out answers to questions they had in tandem with me. I was handed all kinds of "deep books" along with the giver's return addresses, and found myself exchanging names and contact information with people I basically stumbled across or bumped into. And once I started out on the actual trip to Washington State, I found myself enmeshed in conversations in airports along the way and on each plane ride. I instinctively sensed what was happening—this "coincidence is the handiwork of God" pattern—and grew to enjoy each and every second of it, all the while eagerly anticipating the next twist or turn.

After leaving Atlanta I made a stopover in Phoenix (Arizona) where I hung around for a short time to hobnob with family there. My trip continued on with another stop in San Diego to visit another family member. Both of these layovers were punctuated by an influx of people—many strangers—who invariably offered me information or advice, and took a little of my own for themselves.

Arriving in Seattle and catching an inexpensive bus ride to the Greyhound bus station provided its own little adventure insofar as I met yet another a kind spirit who had things to share. From here the bus ride to Wenatchee through the Northern Cascades was quiet and peaceful, memorable mainly because of the beauty that filled my eyes, heart and mind.

At Wenatchee I boarded another little bus that was to carry me to a village named Pateros where Brother Harry was slated to pick me up and get me to Twisp. Here I would spend the night in his home.

The ride with Harry was an interesting mix of driving along precariously narrow roadways at night for about 40 minutes—animated by our ceaseless chitchat. This fellow was more than a little interesting, as he had led a very unusual and different life style than anything I had run across before. Yet I found him to be the most kind and caring individual, full of outward fun and a sense of enjoyment with what he was doing.

The next morning we set off to see the teepee I had heard about, mainly so that I could decide if this is where I wanted to hole up with God and nature. It turned out to be an easy decision, for as we moved up a narrow dirt trail to the top of a Pine tree festooned area, and then glanced back at what had to be one of the most breathtaking views I'd ever see—everything was settled. This was the exact spot to 'screw' back on my head. Peaceful, quiet, serene with a river close by, animals to visit with and the owner of the land living but a short distance away, this was indeed the perfect retreat for this seeker.

Of course, the plan was for me be all alone. Things didn't quite work out that way. The people who took me to this wonderful spot returned the following morning asking if I would help them with some field work. So off I went to work, albeit a bit slowed by my physical infirmities. Surprisingly it felt good even though that night my body was visited by demons of pain.

Many wondrous experiences followed on the heels of that first excruciating day and night—meeting and helping a man who had lost both legs; befriending a young Native American woman and her son; having a light visit me in my "electricity free" teepee during a long, dark night; group meditation sessions; and last but not least, I wound up with answers to the three main questions I came to this retreat with: "What am I supposed to be doing with the rest of my life?" And when I know that—"Where should I be doing this?" And finally, "What am I going to do about money to live on?"

The answers to the questions just "came to me"—however, I did not have any real confidence in what I was hearing in my inner man. I thought it was a joke, and did my best to set them aside and think on other things.

Once I got back home to the sweltering Carolinas, I found myself basically spinning my wheels in neutral. No matter what direction I took, nothing seemed to pan out. Besides that, my body was suffering mightily with the hot, humid weather, and as a result my emotions were on edge. It did not take long for me to quit fighting the inner conviction that the answers that had come to me should be taken seriously. I surrendered myself to what had to be the will of Providence; to return to nature, trees, mountains and the peace that attended them. It was time to be totally open to new experiences and to trusting the Higher Spirit, God!

There were now at least two pressing things I needed to do: One was to hold a yard sale and see about selling off my small stash of surplus goods and such. The other was to get my old 'heap of metal' car, with all of 212,000 miles on it and a body that looked like the junk yard special, worthy of making a cross country trip. Thankfully, a mechanic friend offered to look it over and make it road worthy.

The yard sale came together beautifully and worked like a charm—everything sold the first day. Again, the Universe had jumped in to assist, but only when I had opened up and cooperated. Now I had money to cover all the expenses of making the long trek back to the Pacific Northwest, plus some extra. The only remaining challenge concerned my 'iron horse'. Would the old jalopy be up to this task?

With a sad look in his weathered eyes, my mechanic friend made his diagnosis and gave me the prognosis: "This car will not make it out of the state, let alone coast to coast. Better chuck this idea of an adventure on the Pacific Northwest and stay put."

This bit of bad news fell off my back like water on a Mallard duck. I was now filled with an upbeat, positive attitude and just "knew that I knew that I knew" that my ole body was marching to orders from a higher power. I smiled, thanked the mechanic and even gave him a bear hug to boot for all he had done. I then drove back to my apartment to load up and head out west to continue my quest—my own rendition of 'hide and seek'.

The trip out west found me talking to the old metal heap as though it could understand my every word. Surely she must have turned up a bumper at hearing how trust worthy she was (in my eyes); a good 'Betsy' who would show everyone how she would haul me safely and gently down the highways and back roads across the country to my new home. And lo and behold, "Betsy" not only made the entire trip in one piece and with nary a problem, but continued to serve me well for another 50,000 miles, all without needing anything beyond normal maintenance, i.e., oil changes, tires, fluids, etc. Then when I finally sold ole Betsy, she refused to the honor and promptly "died" on the spot. She found her final resting place in a "junk yard" where some kind soul purchased her carcass and spent many hours and dollars restoring her to full usefulness.

The Holographic Imprint
of a Man in
Verse and Rhyme
© Written by Gloria Shemorry
About Jim Haverlock

My Town ©

My town was near a river running
Slowly south, then east.
I fished and swam and played there
With my friends, my dog,
I'd feast on sandwiches and cookies,

That I'd taken for the day when
Dad's garage got to me
And I could get away.
Sometimes, I'd take a gun along
Pretending I was tall;
Maybe spot a pheasant or a rabbit
That was all;
Until I grew to rifle size stalked antelope
And deer;
I never questioned who I was or
Why God put me here.

CHAPTER FOUR
SPREADING WINGS
WITH A NEW LIFE

Making a home in the Methow Valley and the sweet little, very diverse town of Twisp with its population of 1,000 intrepid souls, several dogs, cats and the huge population of deer was not only relatively easy, but a "good fit" all the way round.

However, when I first got to Twisp I discovered that there were no apartments or rooms of any kind to be found in the region, for they were all taken. Again the Universe stepped in and cleared a path for me. A woman and her male partner had recently opened a real estate office on the main highway through Twisp, suggested that I obtain a real estate license and come work with them. They also had a small studio apartment above the real estate office and offered it to me for a very reasonable rate, including utilities. I could not refuse and moved in within the week.

Moving was easy, as I had come with only what would fit in "Betsy." Thankfully, the owners furnished me with a small table and two plastic lawn chairs. Later on I went to Seattle and discovered all kinds of goodies to be had at local yard and garage sales; things like a futon mattress for the floor, a radio on a cardboard box and a $1.00 lamp to serve as a source of light for reading at night. Yes, it was a humble beginning, but I had a "home" again and it felt so very right.

During my first month on-the-job I studied real estate courses and spent a few hours each day in the real estate office. This was enjoyable and fun and did not even feel like work. In time I made the trek to Seattle to take the real estate agent's exam, passed this, and soon was able to hang out my shingle. Then began the actual work of a selling real estate agent in the valley, learning the roads, the properties for sale, the people, the county and state laws and regulations and as much as I could about other local real estate businesses.

At first I felt like a fish out of water, and worked pretty much part time. I used my abundant free time touring the valley, meeting new friends, traveling to Seattle to see the new friends I had made there, and called on the only relatives I had in the area, a foster son and his wife. Work was not a first priority and the owners were well aware of my "new life style" and did not mind this at all. In fact they encouraged me to be me—which at this stage included sporting "silly bandanas". In some ways, I was living out my own version of the acclaimed TV series "Northern Exposure."

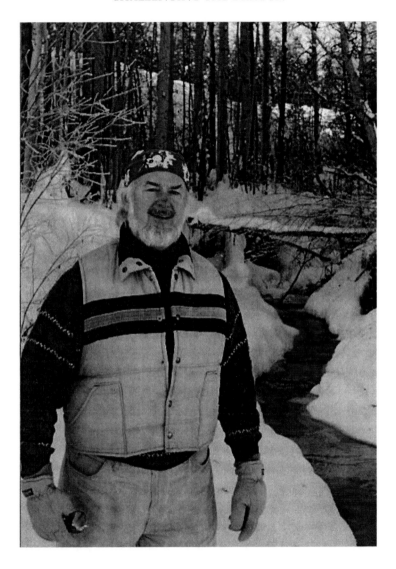

Of course, walk-in clients would stare at this bandana clad, bearded man that greeted them and were often not sure how to react. But within a very few minutes of exchanging niceties, they invariably became comfortable and we wound up having a good time discussing their needs. Then I'd show them properties that suited their tastes and needs, provide necessary information for them to make a decision, all the while being careful to not apply any pressure whatsoever. This helped instill a feeling of being taken care of and not 'rushed' or 'pushed' in everyone I worked for. By not allowing myself to feel pressured by money considerations or ego, I remained cool and calm—which came across to my clients. Learning that what one puts forth, comes back from those around oneself was a most valuable lesson, one not to be forgotten or taken lightly.

Commission real estate agents do not make a dime until a property is sold and the money changes hands. It took two months for me to make a first sale and reap some needed dollars! It was a good thing that my studio apartment costs were low and my life style was very "low maintenance." Actually I learned to live on just $350 per month during that first year— and found it afforded me a minimalist lifestyle that carried with it no stress, worries or surprises. All of my children were on their own to boot and had long ago told me not to worry about them, to just take care of myself and enjoy life. This I did, without reservations of any kind, one day at a time.

During my first winter in Twisp, I discovered that not only nature but human life slows to a snails pace. This provided lots of time to visit new friends, to learn more about valley life and to just be me. Unless one actually witnesses the stark stillness of a white, snow filled winter—a world punctuated only rarely by the sounds of pickup trucks fitted with snow plows moving snow from the driveways and roads, or quail making their morning and evening warning calls—it is impossible to fully appreciate the pervasive sense of peacefulness that attends all this. To sit around a fire with friends, either outside or in a home visiting over a cup of tea or coffee, is a joy unspeakable. Even helping to fix a meal shared by many folks proved a delight; time well spent.

Spring is often likened to a rebirth or a renewing of life. Up in the "Great White North", the snowy surroundings give way to the vibrant colors and hues of life reborn—green grass, shades of green leaves and bushes, the blossoming of yellow balsamroot flowers that filled the mountain sides everywhere. And there was Nature's spring symphony—the morning songs of countless bird species. The sight of new born fawns, quail babies, flowers, gardens popping up from seeds planted after ground frosts are over, and the smiles on all the faces I would see each new day was nourishment for my soul.

I continued to work part time though I gradually added a few more hours, which helped nurture along my mastery of the real estate business. Soon I acquired a few listings of my own and found great joy is seeing them on the local multiple listing service. The owners did all they could to help me learn the inner workings of the business, as well as the Methow Valley area we serviced.

The Valley itself is narrow and long and surrounded by state and federal lands on all sides, leaving little private land for sale. The sheer "smallness" of this parcel of terra firma combined with the splendor of the land itself enhanced its appeal to big city people seeking a "escape" in the country. Lookers, as we called them, flooded the office in spring, summer and fall seeking their "piece of heaven" and finding prices that were typically well beyond their means. A real estate agent can show properties to a great many people before finding the few that can afford and really want a specific property.

By the following winter I found myself looking at a

real estate office that was for sale in the vicinity. It was not maintained properly, mainly because the owner spent most of his time working a little hay farm and no longer had a lot of interest in real estate sales. As a consequence, the listings were down to just 4 or 5 and sales were pretty much non-existent. I found the whole thing a challenge and an opportunity, so I stepped out and made the owner an offer. We haggled and then agreed on a price. As part of the bargain, he agreed to remain on as broker until I obtained my broker's license. We then closed the deal and I now had my own real estate office!

In short order my new business grew and I found myself taking on a young female agent, as well as a young man wanting to work part time. More growth found me hiring yet another agent, whose family belonged to the old time valley residents. Soon our listing file grew to over 130 listings.

People seeking property, homes or buildings liked our down home honesty and our "treat them as you'd want to be treated" policy. This was actually an understood priority in our office and it paid off handsomely in terms of generating both revenue and goodwill. Not surprisingly, in a market that consisted of eleven real estate offices and some 60 agents, we went from being number 11 to being number 4 within our first year of operation.

All was not bliss however. I had my share of "trouble in Paradise", mainly in the form of physical ability losses that continued to wreak havoc on this body, including difficulty walking, balance and speech. Within a couple of years it became evident that I could not continue to show property, especially the 20 and 40 acre lots that required walking about extensively. Realizing my limitations, I decided to merge my office with another down the road and continue working only part time as an associate broker.

During this period of being a real estate "tycoon", I also had time to take advantage of the many adventures that the valley provides, like hiking and sightseeing. Looking beyond the Valley, Washington State was rich with opportunities to explore: Among these are the Pacific Ocean and Puget Sound, the mountains and valleys, desert areas, orchards galore and then farm lands that go on for miles, the many rivers and streams, and a wealth of tree and birth species. One could, in fact, spend an entire lifetime touring this state and not see the same things twice.

I also made a point of traveling beyond Washington State's borders, to points-of-interest within the US, Canada and the world at large. Though I had been repeatedly advised by my doctors not to travel alone, this "flyin' blind" guy did it anyway. I took 10 weeks off and traveled alone to Germany where I spent fourteen days with friends, then paid a second visit to the Nieper clinic in Hanover. This was followed by jaunts to Bangkok and on to Singapore where I stayed for a week with friends of my foster son and his wife.

Then I pressed on to Kuching, Malaysia to stay with my foster son's wife's family for a few weeks. They showed me around the area, taught me to enjoy new foods, and I even grew to appreciate the hot, humid weather that characterized this equatorial country. I especially enjoyed spending time milling around among the local people, and came to admire how they could live on what seemed so little and be so very happy. Their gentleness and genuine smiles were not lost on me either.

I was fortunate to see the world's largest flower which only grows in one area of Malaysia (near Borneo) and to say it is huge is an understatement! The world's largest flower, the 'rafflesia' measuring up to a metre across, looks artificial because of its sheer gargantuan dimensions, but it is every bit real. Following this, a local native wanted me to accompany him to the top of a nearby mountain; one that had to be reached by primitive roads part way and then a trail. I agreed and wound up spending the day in an area inhabited only by monkeys, snakes and other wild creatures. Nature had some other surprises, too, such as some heavy rain that hit us as we ascended this mostly un-traveled mountain. We were a sight, sliding in mud until we both thought we would slide off and take the quick way down—into the abyss below. It was dark and still raining when we finally decided that turning back was the greater part of valor. By the time we got back to Kuching, we were both starving and ready to chow down on some good ole home cooking—so we used my companion's cell phone to let his family know we were homeward bound. Of course, family had a fantastic meal waiting for us upon our arrival.

Next I was off to Kuala Lumpur for a few days, then back to Singapore for a couple more, then on to Frankfort, Germany where I was to catch my flight back to the states. However, once I got to Germany I discovered that my flight was overbooked by 70 seats. So were ALL the flights to the states for the next several days. With my funds now running low, hanging around was a bad idea. I had to find a way home.

While standing in line at the airline counter, I struck up a conversation with another chap anxious to get home and we wound up becoming friends of a sort. Again the Universe was moving in strange ways, for this man had been on a photographic assignment in Russia for the past couple of months and he was anxious to get back to San Francisco and his home.

As we chatted about what to do, we hit upon checking flights from Paris. We did this and found seats available for the next morning. We booked our respective flights out of Paree,

bought train tickets from Frankfort to Paris and hit the road—
or the tracks.

We arrived in Paris late at night, walked to the nearest
hotel, booked a shared room and promptly fell asleep. Waking
early we made our way to the subway station where we caught
a train to the airport and arrived in time to catch our flight to
New York City. We said our goodbyes at the airport in NYC
and went in different directions and back to our respective
homes. We did stay in touch for a time although we have not
seen one another since.

Later on I made a trip to North Carolina to visit family,
than a month later found myself returning there for my
father's funeral. He lived to the ripe old age of 93, leaving fond
memories galore for me to relive down through the years. Two
years later my mother passed on and I once more made by way
to North Carolina to take part in the funeral proceedings and
to be with siblings.

Spreading my wings by taking on the real estate venture
full bore and then traveling was both fulfilling and rewarding.
It gave me courage, hope and a sense of being productive and
adventurous in spite of my physical challenges. It was a time
of rebirth for me just like every winter gives way to Nature's
annual rebirth each spring. And it provided me the opportunity
to meet so many new people, to make a whole host of new
friends and to get to really know the valley which I now called
"home". It also reminded me that I could and did still take
falls—anywhere—anytime—including faraway exotic locales
in Germany, Bangkok, Singapore, Malaysia, and France.

Que sie ra, sie ra—whatever will be, will be.

CHAPTER FIVE
MOVING ON
COMPUTER AND INTERNET

Being involved in the world of real estate was, and is, a very interesting and enjoyable line of business. I especially enjoyed meeting so many new and wonderful people, and the good feeling knowing I have helped assist them in finding their dream property or home or office. However, the time came to "let go" of this business and move on, mainly due to my "challenged" life style. It is often very difficult to admit to oneself something family and friends have seen for some time, but there comes a time for facing realty. Being a stubborn person, this process took me much longer, something not so surprising when you consider the fact I smoked for 20 years before admitting this was unhealthy and then quitting. My approach to quitting smoking pretty much reflected how I square off when recognizing a problem and then dealing with it: I typically use no aids, just sheer stubbornness and self determination.

Being the sort of fellow who looks forward to trying challenging new things, I found the world of computers a natural. I had first made the acquaintance of PCs in my real estate work and actually became adept at using it to get things done. At first, I and my office crew kept an inventory of our listings using database software. Then we began creating and printing out brochures on each property using another form of software designed for that purpose. The local realtors formed our own multiple listing service (MLS) and we all wound up joining the now expanding internet. With the assistance of a friend, I learned how to build web sites and then built one for showing our listings and also as a tool to promote our clients' properties. Within two years I became the president of our local MLS.

As the showing of properties had become increasingly difficult for my body, turning to the computer was a very natural fallback. Actually, it was the best choice I could make—as it enabled me to continue to feel productive, provided a needed challenge for my mind and soul, and gave an outlet for the frustration of "giving in" or "letting go" of another portion of life as I knew it.

At first I did odd jobs for others like making brochures, scanning pictures, building simple little web sites and such. As I became more comfortable with the software and technology, I branched into building a web site for the many people who wanted to sell property on their own, without paying the high costs of a real estate agency and its commission fees.

With a computer-oriented career now clearly set in my mind as a goal, I set about studying, researching and learning more about computers, the internet and the World Wide Web. It wasn't long before the new web site started taking shape along with ideas of how to promote it, both to gain clients and to promote their listings. Both of these were key needs in making this new venture a success.

Meantime, I continued to work part time as a real estate agent and also managed a mini storage facility for its owner. I even took up living in an apartment at the storage facility, which allowed me ample time to play with the computer and step up my learning curve. It wasn't long before the new site was up and running, giving this "challenged" soul a feeling of fitting into the "normal world" again. The domain name and URL for this site became http://AbetterFSBO.com which stood for "A Better For Sale By Owner ".

It wasn't long before I realized that there were hundreds of other people in the world also running "fsbo" advertising sites. Competition was and is everywhere, even the internet!!

My website project was working well enough but just didn't provide enough revenue to make ends meet. While thinking about this venture, mainly my lack of sufficient income, another thought occurred. What about the furniture business? I had many years experience running furniture stores, selling on the road to other stores, working with factories all over the USA, so why not build an "online furniture outlet"? Why not indeed!

My main dilemma now was how to begin going about this. Rhetorical questions now began racing through my mind: How about starting with a list of the factories I am familiar with? Then creating another list including all of the factory representatives that I know? And another sheet with a list of ideas on how to build such a business, long term and short term goals and all of the ideas on how to reach this goal? These were the seeds for the revenue machine I envisioned.

After putting these thoughts down on paper, I then called up an old friend in the furniture business to discuss the idea. Over the years I had learned that "talking" with others provided answers much more readily then just sitting and thinking up things on one's own. Sure enough, this friend represented a factory selling bar stools and he quickly volunteered to contact them and get permission to add me as a dealer selling online.

The excitement that comes with a new idea and its implementation reminds me of how our space program came to be. First came fantasies expressed in books, then dreaming aloud about the possibilities, the grunt work of putting ideas down on paper and then testing them out with small scale model rockets, then larger and grander experiments, until finally not just machines or animals but men were being lifted into the heavens.

To my way of thinking, I was a NASA unto myself and was about to launch into high orbit. Although my feat was not as risky as putting one's life on the line, I was still vesting badly needed time and money on a calculated gamble. Money?! This was a challenge indeed, because I only had my small disability income, and not much coming in anymore from the real estate business. Mine was a thin shoestring indeed!

While waiting for an answer from my friend concerning permission from the furniture factory to become an online dealer, something I was convinced would come to pass, I started seeking ways to build this online venture from scratch. It would be necessary to learn much more about html language, the language used to build the most visually appealing and user friendly kind of web pages. Of course, I also had to set up a FAX number and a phone service for people to use in calling in orders, and settle on payment options.

And there was Uncle Sam to contend with: I needed a software accounting system to keep records, not only tracking orders and payments, but also to keep the Internal Revenue Service and the State Tax Department happy.

All of this work had to be accomplished without any large money backers, with no investment capital—only an idea and a prayer. Truly a "flying blind" type of adventure, one that this writer is all too familiar with!

Quiet, StillnessTo live!

By Jim Haverlock ©

Making a living, the bills to pay,
Working hard throughout the day.
Evening finds this tired old back and 'ass'
Horizontal on this earth's lovely grass.
Gazing towards the heavenly skies
These weary and droopy old eyes,
Watching lazily the clouds slowly drift
Making a myriad of shapes a lovely gift
The birds overhead do swiftly glide
'Nary a care they joyously sing and ride
Still closer to this body on the ground do fly
God's little winged creatures, oh my!
Turning over I gaze at the ground
Interspersed with busy ants all around
The sun slowly setting in the west
Every one now heads towards their nest
Like a child with an inquisitive mind.
This oldster turns childish in kind
Time for many thanks the Maker to give,
Especially for quiet, stillness, to live!

As was my habit, I plowed into study, research, learning and then "trial & (lots of) error" implementation all what I was slowly mastering. Slowly but surely I tooled together a web site, all the while keeping my ear cocked for the phone to ring with news that I had been approved as a dealer and would then be given pictures, price lists and descriptions of the products.

The phone call I was looking for did come at last and was a "thumbs up". The furniture company people indicated that they knew me and my situation, and were more than willing to give this a go. A catalog of their products along with descriptions, pricing and pictures would be expressed to me pronto. It was T minus 10 seconds and counting—almost time for "blast off." Now the real work is about to begin.

Once the catalog arrived, I painstakingly scanned in pictures and resized them to fit the allotted space on my website. Web pages were built to display each product, its description, the options available and finally, the pricing for each item. I also set about creating an online form that would accommodate anticipated orders, as well as trying to make sure my web address would pop up whenever folks used a major search engine like Google (www.google.com) to hunt down furniture.

The day finally arrived when all of the details and grunt work were finished and my web site could at last be transferred to the server, who would then place my brainchild out there in cyber-space for anyone with access to the internet to find. It was now lift off time!

And what a thrill it was when I accessed the new site for the first time! There it was on my computer screen, my new store front—in all its glory—http://www.14ushop.com. To my way of thinking, it was the most gorgeous store front ever! I had achieved orbit!

The joy found in being creative, of seeing one's thoughts and ideas become a reality, is difficult to express in terms others who've not "been there" can readily appreciate. In some ways, I think what I felt then and still feel must be in some way akin to what women feel when they have their first child: A heady mix of pain, pleasure, joy and fear

Of course, it was no small consolation that my dream was a bridge to self-sufficiency; a means to be productive in the "normal world".

My journey to self-sufficiency was by no means easy for this "challenged" body. The daily difficulties that come with multiple sclerosis present one with hurdle after hurdle after hurdle to negotiate. For those of you who do not have MS, or who do not know someone with this "challenge", here are but a few of the obstacles and bumps in the road that can crop up as a result of the disease process:

Let's start with eyesight. Many people with MS find their eye sight in a state of continual flux, changing many times throughout the day. This is my case and the glasses I wear and use are of much help, but not the answer that "normal" people find to be true. Blurred vision occurs when least expected or wanted.

Fatigue comes into play almost every day too. Fortunately my fatigue level is pretty good considering for a person with progressive MS. Many times at the end of a work day I find my old body not quite willing to prepare a meal, or tend to the house cleaning chores that beckon, or even head over to visit a friend. Instead, I find myself just wanting to get horizontal and let the cares of the world float on by. But with so much that needs doing, I invariably have to grab myself by the seat of the pants and swing into high gear. Anything less is giving in to the Dragon, which I will not do.

Dexterity is an issue for most "challenged" people, and I am no exception, although more fortunate again then others. Typing for hours on end is a good exercise in terms of maintaining my manual dexterity, which comes in handy for picking up small objects. If I didn't keep this faculty honed, manipulating tiny items would surely become a real nightmare!

Of course, getting from one spot in the office to another is yet another task to conquer on a regular basis; one that takes thought, consideration and then making it happen. And while wheel chairs or power chairs are tremendous assets when getting about easily on one's own is difficult or impossible, it isn't easy to give up stumbling about for wheeling about.

Then there is the matter of my speech, which MS causes to be slurred somewhat like what you'd hear from someone who'd spent an entire night tossing back drink after drink. This, of course, makes being understood by people who call me up on the phone a bit intimidating. Actually, this is the biggest frustration for me, as I love conversing with the people who call up my business to place orders; many of whom call in from exotic locales all over the world. Having people hang up on me is not uncommon. It has happened often enough actually such that phone calls are now routinely taken by members of my small staff. Missing out on having a conversation with someone in another part of the world—especially in countries I've visited—are a thing of the past, and another "death to mourn".

There are other issues and hurdles common to people with my particular "challenge", and each case is unique and the symptoms are as varied and diverse as people afflicted. It is my belief that no two people with MS manifest it exactly in the same way, and with there being several hundred thousand people with MS, there are just as many variations in symptoms.

Families touched by MS also face a wealth of challenges—physically, mentally, emotionally, and spiritually. Many family members and friends find it much easier to never talk about it, to avoid the "victim", and in some instances do not accept it or only partially do so. This inability or unwillingness to confront

MS is a familiar theme, for we who have the condition all have family members and/or close friends who choose not to stay in contact because of it. The saddest part of this is that they are very much needed. Yes, MS is a journey that family members and friends are not obligated to grapple with. They need only accept us the way we are and for who we are. We do not, and have not, changed; only our bodies—our Earthsuits—have. The "real person" continues on, though its trappings and frame are peeling and dilapidated and thus in need of some tender loving care. At times MS seems like an antiquated prison or medieval dungeon, dark and musty and in need of visits from friends bearing candles!

This reminds me of a letter written by a famous man who helped found this country (I believe this was Thomas Jefferson), to his best friend, it goes something like this:

"The house I live in is becoming dilapidated. The roof has become bare, the windows are dull and dim, the very walls have become weak and their strength is gone. Yes, this house is becoming dilapidated and soon I shall have to leave it. But, I am well."

This final letter depicts his body as the house he lives in—but he is "well". I like that analogy, it is one I believe true also.

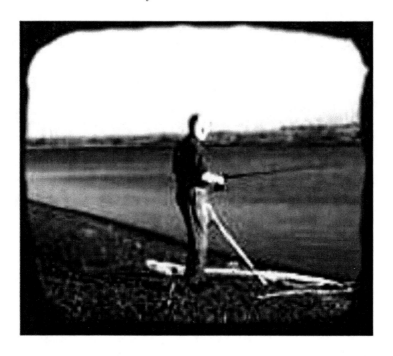

A 'TRUE' North Dakota

FISH STORY

With MS, you always wonder about last times...the last time you ran on the beach, the last time you flew a plane (If you're a private pilot like me), the last time you engaged in a recreational sport—like fishing in my case. In my new home there was no beach—I wasn't "fit" to fly—so this left fishing. And as it had been about 14 years since I had been fishing, and despite the fact my balance wasn't good enough to walk without a cane, I was determined to hold a rod and reel in hand again. So late on afternoon I went down to the Missouri River with a brand new 6 ft. rod and spinning reel from Wal-Mart and the few lures that came with the combo unit in-hand.

My casting was a little rusty before long I was sending the life-like minnow flying a considerable distance into the river, than retrieving it with a flare. Not bad for a man who had to prop himself up with a cane! The downside was that I was not catching anything! One always hopes for a big strike on the first few casts, but this wasn't the case. So I cast some more but again, no fish. That went on for about ten tries, then a friend who'd come along with me tried his hand at it.

With a self-assured style, he cast out a considerable distance and, then began the retrieval. He took his share of casting turns (actually more than his share) then handed the rod to me, and I attached my favorite red and white daredevil lure. A few more turns and we tried the squiggly squid, a diving fluorescent bottom feeder...even a green wiggly worm. This went on for about two hours, with not so much as a strike. We did, however, bring in several broken tree limbs, which we reverently released back into the river.

It was such a glorious day that we actually didn't mind the lack of interest on the part of the fish. The sky was blue, the sun was shining brightly and a huge flock of Mallard ducks was "heckling" us. Their incessant chatter actually made us laugh all afternoon long. And we had visitors too. Two men riding their 4-wheel ATV's came up looking for an easy spot to climb up off the river bank. It turned out one of them was an old friend of mine and, of course, we had a nice "catch-up" visit after what had been a 15 year absence.

About 5:30 pm, my friend decided to head back to the house and get dinner going, allowing me to have full control of the fishing expedition. Thankfully he left the truck so I wouldn't have to walk the few hundred yards back to the house. I was about finished up with fishing too, but upon my third and "last" cast of the day, a 'monster' fish attacked my red and white daredevil lure! What a thrill—to feel that tug on the line, the whir of the line leaving the reel, and the thought of showing off my 'catch' to my friend.

Of course, the "catch to this catch" lay in the fact that I had poor balance and could not stand too long without the use of at least one cane. And here I was, standing with a cane propped against my body, handle in my lower tummy area, the other end pushed into the soft mud, trying to balance myself while reeling in whatever had latched onto my bait.

Not surprisingly the fish was not complying with my game plan, and I was getting nowhere near bringing him closer to shore. My reel was set with sufficient tension to bring in a 3 to 4 pound fish—but this one was pulling line out from the reel with ease! After a couple of minutes, I managed to tighten the tension a 'wee' bit so as not to cause the 8 lb line to break from the strain of battle that was now raging on.

In time I managed to bring the 'monster' fish in a few feet closer, than it took off to the right—pulling the line out again. And again I brought it in closer, and then it took off to the left, pulling line from the reel with what seemed like effortless ease. Although I was getting tired (not just from fighting the fish, but from trying to keep upright), I managed to adjust the tension one more time.

My legs were getting wobbly, my hands and wrists were definitely tiring, but the thought of bringing a really big one home kept me going. Where was my friend when I needed him? Thanks to the MS, I couldn't holler anymore, and I knew that I would just have to do this alone—and if I didn't bring this fish in, he'd never believe my tale. The sound of "heckling" from the ever present Mallards drove this home in spades.

After about 20 minutes of give-and-take the fish began to tire, and I began to think of the next big hurdle—how I would get this thing out of the water without losing it! And if I cleared this hurdle, how did I propose picking it up and hauling it to the house? (Retrieving anything from the floor is only done with great difficulty even when there are things to lean on.) In any event, I was beginning to realize there was more involved here than getting the big strike.

Finally, the fish was almost on shore, when the rod, which was bent almost double under the weight and pressure of this monster, snapped and broke off! Now the fish really had an advantage over me. Great! I let go of the spinning handle, grabbed my cane and—using the tip—managed to maneuver the fish ashore. The line then broke causing me to almost lose my balance. Again, I dragged the fish further on shore with my cane. Then using the cane to balance myself, I slowly bent over and stuck my fingers in the gill and lifted it up. But my miniature Leviathan wasn't through fighting and flipped in mid-air and fell back to the ground in a desperate attempt to beat a hasty return to the water. Balancing myself with the cane, I grabbed the fish again, fingers securely in the gills and somehow managed to get it up into the back of the pickup truck. My friend would believe me for sure now. 'Proof 'was in-hand.

My friend's eyes lit up as he headed out toward the truck and got his first glimpse of this monster fish. "Holy cow, its huge", he exclaimed. We both looked the fish over thoroughly, admiring its size and fortitude. It was a huge carp—about 12-14 pounds, and although exhausted from it's well fought battle with me, it was still very much alive, even if it was on dry land.

Supper was already ready cooking on the stove, and the fish would represent "overkill" if added to all this. It seemed a shame to kill him anyway, so we decided to give him another chance. He was still hanging on to life when we placed him in the water. Now back in his native habitat he began to slowly recover. When we were sure he was going to make it, we eased him out into the deeper water, and watched as he disappear into the depths. Despite the egg rolls and green salad we had for dinner that night, our spirits were warmed by the one that didn't get away. And I had the thrill of a lifetime, knowing that there might still be a few more catches in life in store for me

CHAPTER SIX
MOURNING LOSSES

A "nose down, tail spin" mix of emotions is a natural consequence of losing something vital. No doubt most of those reading my words have experienced loss in the past. Maybe you lost a dog, cat or pet fish as a child, or you might remember the loss of a "first love," or lost friends when they moved away. Many experience the loss of important relationships through death, separation or divorce. With Multiple Sclerosis you are often confronted with the loss of a productive life as well as any dreams of achieving a viable future.

"Death is the least of my worries. I always knew it would happen someday. But it's watching part of me die each day that is so terrifying."

Mine are primarily losses of the flesh. Your losses may be different. You may not have the energy or spirit to function well as a parent, spouse, or friend. You may not have the strength to work or pursue activities you once enjoyed. You may often want to be alone.

Medications may make you very tired. You may be alone because family and friends begin to distance themselves, in part as a way to cope with their own loss. It is then that you will realize that life is propelling you to the finish line over the roughest terrain you could ever have imagined. Can you recover from the changes and disappointments? To survive the "little deaths" we must be able to mourn each loss as it occurs.

In spite of what society suggests or well-intentioned friends offer, mourning is a normal, healthy response to loss. It helps us to survive all kinds of troubles, so that we can make necessary adjustments to change. It's generally easier to mourn for another and perhaps a bit self-indulgent to mourn for yourself, but letting yourself do so can be healing for body, mind and soul.

What's especially important, I've discovered, is that we all find a way to mourn that ultimately brings some degree of comfort.

With MS, the need to grieve for one's losses (in whatever way is comfortable) will recur at different times as the "challenge" unfolds. Death becomes not a single event but a succession of smaller ones leading up to the fatal blow. "I find that every time my body lets me down or I see myself getting sicker, I become inconsolable. I wish that I could go to my cave and disappear." (As the book "Men are from Mars, Women are from Venus" said—men run to their caves—that is me for sure.)

Crying can be a good way to mourn the "little deaths." Other ways can be just as effective. It is finding one that works, that helps one to cope that is the most important thing.

I felt sorry for myself and did a little mourning over these injuries suffered because of my determination to live life to the fullest, and have the scars to show for it.

- Broken ribs (2 first time, 3 the next and same 3 again)
- Many shin injuries, too many to count
- Head injuries from falling backwards (not able to stop them) one of which people who witnessed the fall, saw all the blood, knew I was unconscious, they

drove away leaving me to crawl to the car, drive into Twisp and seek some help.

- Concussions—4—one 911 was called, one neighbors hauled me unconscious to hospital, one in Canada (someone got me to the hospital where I awoke) Yikes!
- Torn Rotator Cuff—twice—surgery had to be performed—95% use back
- Cracked vertebrae in spine—falling in bath tub
- Broken rib by spine (back)—falling against bath tub
- More banged and cut fingers and toes then can count

CHAPTER SEVEN
WHEN THE GOING GETS TOUGH

B ig boys don't cry!"
"Only babies cry, stop it!"
"No pain, no gain."
"Life is tough so toughen up!"

"There is nothing wrong with you. You're only looking for attention."

The first four sentences are comments hurled at me during the early years of my life, one's I am sure most of us have heard many times over. They were meant to "toughen" us up to the real world, right?

The very last phrase in the litany above is one my father expressed when I accidentally fell in my parents' apartment. "There is nothing wrong with you. You're only looking for attention." This was difficult to hear—and just as difficult to share now. Yet it is a part of my life.

I wound up spending the better part of a year trying to explain to my parents the nature of my illness, and thought they understood. They knew how my life had changed, that my wife had left me right after I was diagnosed, and that the business I was part owner of at the time was stolen out from under me. Yet my father would not accept what was happening—or did not want to. His dismissive, almost flippant statement is one I've forgiven him for repeatedly in my heart, however the words remain seared into my memory and constitutes one of the worst hurts I ever endured.

For me, the going got toughest in the wake of family and friends who would not, or could not face the reality of my situation. It is an understandable, although hurtful fact of life and of human nature to deny reality and chose avoidance. It is natural, yes, but not fair.

Coming to grips with the diagnosis was not easy for me, and I am sure that most of the people with this diagnosis would say the same thing was true of them when they received their "medical sentence." Who really wants to grapple with the fact that life will never be the same again? Who wants to consider the possibility of losing their independence? Who wants to face having a spouse or loved one walk away? Who wants to face losing their productivity? Mobility? Speech? Eyesight? Or having to contemplate a future day in which someone may have to "wipe your butt?"

None of these nasty possibilities are acceptable. One's reaction is outrage—and a desire to run and hide. But to have others tell you there is nothing wrong with you, that you are just seeking attention, is even more hurtful then the cruel disease itself.

When the going got really tough for me—is when I turned to the only place left to turn: God, the creator, the higher being, the all knowing, the all seeing, the "I AM". Like a child in pain, yelling for "Mom" with just one word, I found myself screaming "HELP!" It is surely the simplest of prayers, but effective—for "mom" ran in and soothed the pain.

Unlike some saddled who wrestle with my particular dragon, I never blamed God. Everything on this planet that lives experiences peaks and valleys including sickness, then one day dies and moves on. Why should it be any different for me? It wasn't part of any plan I would ever conceive, nor something

I wanted or chose to have. But it was the hand I had been dealt and my only choice was to play it out.

We all have choices as to how we live our life, with or without an added challenge such as MS. Granted it is more difficult to make a choice when faced with a prolonged, especially incurable disease or "challenge". Illness and debility is indeed a lot tougher road to journey down, but many folks like myself are plunked down on it and must make the trek. So why not choose to do it with a smile, helping others along the way? And do the best one can with what resources one can muster, never giving up hope, but always seeking ways to improve not only one's own lot but that of others? Perhaps our losses help or inspire others without our even knowing it.

A Walk through Life

I've learned—
that you can do something in an instant that will give you heartache for life.

I've learned—
that it's taken me a long time to become the person I want to be.

I've learned—
that you should always leave loved ones with loving words. It may be the last time you see them.

I've learned—
that you can keep going long after you can't.

I've learned—
that we are responsible for what we do, no matter how we feel.

I've learned—that either you control your attitude or it controls you.

I've learned—

that regardless of how hot and steamy a relationship is at first, the passion fades and there had better be something else to take its place.

I've learned—

that heroes are the people who do what has to

be done when it needs to be done, regardless of opposition.

I've learned—

that money is a lousy way of keeping score.

I've learned—

that my best friend and I can do anything or nothing and have a great time.

I've learned—

that sometimes the people you expect to kick you when you're down will be the ones to help you get back up.

I've learned—

that sometimes when I'm angry I have the right to be angry, but that doesn't give me the right to be cruel.

I've learned—

that true friendship continues to grow, even over long distance. The same goes for true love.

I've learned—

that just because someone doesn't love you the way you want them to, doesn't mean they don't love you with all they have.

I've learned—

that maturity has more to do with what types of experiences you've had and what you've learned

from them and less to do with how many birthdays you've celebrated.

I've learned—

that your family won't always be there for you. It may

seem ironic, but people you aren't related to often can take care of you and love you and teach you to trust people again when blood kin won't or can't. Families aren't just biological.

I've learned—

that no matter how good a friend is, they're going to hurt you every once in a while and you must forgive them for that.

I've learned—

that it isn't always enough to be forgiven by others, Sometimes you have to learn to forgive yourself.

I've learned—

that our background and circumstances may have influenced who we are, but we are responsible for who we become.

I've learned—

that just because two people argue, it doesn't mean they don't love each other. And just because they don't argue, it doesn't mean they do.

I've learned—

that we don't have to change friends if we understand that friends change.

I've learned—

that you shouldn't be so eager to find out a hidden secret, because it could change your life forever.

I've learned—

that two people can look at the exact same thing and see something totally different.

I've learned—

that your life can be changed in a matter of minutes, by people who don't even know you.

I've learned—

that even when you think you have no more to give, when a friend cries out to you, you will find the strength to help.

I've learned—

that credentials on the wall do not make you a decent human being.

I've learned—

that the people you care about most in life are taken from you too soon.

Author unknown

CHAPTER EIGHT
I. The Alexander Technique

Among the many valuable lessons life taught me was that most of us are blissfully unaware of habits that cause us stress and complicate our ability to cope effectively. In my case, having "Progressive MS" for the past 12+ years has drastically changed my posture and functional mobility. As my nervous system has deteriorated, I developed many maladaptive habits to compensate for lost functions. Thankfully I found a solution in something called "The Alexander Technique". It is a form of mind-body training that is not just for ailing people like me, but also for men and women whose daily grind takes a toll on their bodies.

The technique itself is all about changing maladaptive habits so one can respond more effectively and achieve better, more efficient functioning. Although not well known, the Alexander Technique has been acknowledged by many health care pros for over 100 years as constituting a unique and remarkably effective technique for reeducating one's body.

I am not sure if the inventor of this technique ever meant it for people suffering with M.S., but I can personally attest that it is one of the very few therapies (including drug therapies) that has visibly improved the quality of my life.

Readers who make use of the Internet should visit www. alexandertechnique.com. This particular cyber-education stop is serviced by Robert and Anne Rickover ("Complete Guide to the Alexander Technique.") Robert is an Alexander Teacher among many credentials he possesses in this remarkable, effective healing arts method.

For me, M.S. set the stage for poor posture and with this trouble with balance, walking, sitting, etc. And I was totally unaware that this could be changed and just assumed it was all part of the M.S. experience. When I first heard about the Alexander Technique and was told it might reverse some of my physical losses, I immediately enrolled for private sessions with Josette Pelletier, a certified practitioner.

Once I got into doing the Alexander Technique, I found that unlearning my old MS habits was more than a little challenging, but immensely rewarding—not only in terms of my ability to move and function more efficiently, but also in terms of experiencing the first physical improvements in many years of gradual and progressive decline.

Josette graduated in 1990 from the Pacific Institute of the Alexander Technique in Chico, California, and is currently teaching in Chelan, WA. She is also a massage practitioner and an Hauna-Somatie Instructor. This is what she had to say about working with me.

"My working with Jim has been a wonderful experience that has taught me a great deal. My trust in the workings of the technique is even greater and has shown in this case, to be helpful in reawakening the connection of mind (thought) to the better working of the body."

"When I first met Jim, he walked in with the help of a cane in a slow, contracted way. His joints appeared stiff and flexing with great effort. His upper body compensated with the imbalance with much muscular tension and his speech was slower than normal."

"What struck me about Jim was his honesty, his acceptance

of this limitation, his strength in continuing to trust that he could improve; his willingness to create a strong connection of mind—body communication and lastly that he didn't expect a miracle cure."

"After 13 sessions and Jim's great perseverance in applying the newly learned information, he has a wonderful, re-established balance creating an open and relaxed upper body. His ankles, knees and hips are now moving with much more freedom and he can stand and walk for long periods of time without his cane. It continues to improve bringing more assurance, more energy, less pain, more trust! Certainly his quality of life has improved a great deal!"

Learning the Alexander Technique

What one learns in Alexander Technique lessons is a unique and practical means of identifying, stopping and then changing bad habits. This learning process allows one's sense of coordination to regain its natural form.

Pelletier took me through basic movements giving gentle hands-on guidance. This hands-on education helped me experience more natural, easy coordinated movements without interference from old maladaptive habits. By consistently doing these natural exercises I managed to "reprogram" my internal coordination system so that it became more "real life" again. This helped me reach a point whereby I could choose better coordinated and non-stressful responses to life's daily grind.

BENEFITS

Among the more notable benefit of doing the Alexander Technique or method is that I now stand straighter, taller and have overall better posture. Friends have noticed this change and comment about "how healthy" I look. In addition, my reeducated body now gets into and out of a chair without much ado, something not true prior to my treatments. I also have a better sense of balance and can actually walk short distances without the use of a cane or other support.

II. FAMILY CONSTELLATIONS

"A workshop for those who can trust that solutions may be simple and happen in a short period of time—like stepping from shadow into light..."

Based on the work of Bert Hellinger.

I first heard about "Family Constellations" from my Alexander Teacher and after a few discussions decided to take in a "demo" evening session put on by Brigitte Sztab of Chelan, WA. Being a bit of a skeptic, I attended this session with my guard up.

After informing Brigitte that I was attending to observe, not participate and not to call on me,....*I was selected by another participant to be involved in the first constellation.* Again, the universe was determining the direction of my life, and it was incumbent on me to be open and accepting.

The person doing the work was asked to select people in attendance to represent members of her family that were involved in her issues. Everything was done with the feeling of love, no pressure, no forcing, just being open to the issues. What ensued was utterly amazing. With Brigitte as the leader and guide for this process, events unfolded that made it clear to the participants the origins of the issues being dredged up. Presumably, once you are armed with this knowledge, healing can begin.

Unlike paying an hourly fee to a counselor who typically prescribes many high priced sessions, this work is done during a weekend workshop for one low fee.

According to Brigitte (www.familyconstellations-usa.com) "Family Constellations" is a highly effective way of bringing about healing on a deeply felt energetic level, with long-term and often life changing results.

The system or approach itself was spawned by German psychotherapist Bert Hellinger. In working with several thousand family systems, Hellinger discovered age-old, hidden "Orders of Love" that operate in the depths of family "organisms." Violation and disrespect of these natural laws due to tragic circumstances and unconscious behavior that is transmitted across the generations affects the lives of everyone in the family line.

For instance, according to FC proponents, unhappiness or health problems could be connected, for example, to a stillborn child of a grandmother. Difficulties with one's current partner could be related to an abortion that happened years ago to a near relative.

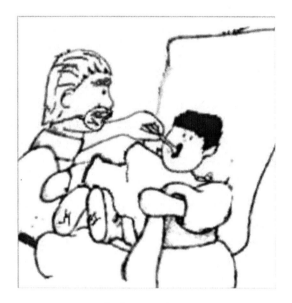

Baby Teeth ©

"This won't hurt,"
he said,
"open wide"
Like a young deer
Too scared to bleet,
I submitted.
From a distance,
I heard
My tooth
Clunking against
The pan.
His face leered
Down from above
"You were a

brave little soldier
and didn't cry,"
he cajoled, adding,
"That wasn't so bad,
was it?"
My eyes sought the floor
For answers, but
It offered none;
Searching, I looked
Up to discover pride
In my mother's eyes.
It was enough.

Hidden entanglements of this kind are found behind most personal and even professional issues. According to advocates, restoring balance and harmony to the family system will be as effective for physical illness—from lower back pain to cancer—as it is for emotional and mental suffering. Family Constellation adroitly reveals them.

Release toward resolution begins with disclosure of a participant's issue or problem and some factual information about his/her family (i.e. sudden or early deaths, severe illness, miscarriage, divorce, etc.).Following this, she chooses a representative for each family member (living or dead) from the other participants—and defines their relationship one to the other according to her inner picture of the family system. This creates an energy field in which all the participants begin to receive information (physical sensations, emotions, thoughts, etc.) related to the family member whom they represent. Every change in position within the constellation affects the information received. As a result, previously sub-conscious, often tragic family ties are made perceptible and the dynamic that caused the participant's issue can be discovered.

With information provided by the representatives, and using steps such as appreciation or detachment, the constellation can now be restructured according to the "Orders of Love" into a balanced family system where love, flowing consciously and unimpeded, heals, and guilt, once acknowledged, can turn into energy.

Family Constellation workshops are designed for individuals and couples interested in solving serious issues, relieving suffering and finding a solid foundation for new direction in their lives. It is also utilized by therapists, psychiatrists, nurses, social workers, physicians and other health care professionals interested in enriching their practice with highly effective tools and new insights about disease, individual issues and human behavior.

During the workshops, participants can and often do:

1. Resolve misunderstandings, entanglements and blocks in family-, partner—and other relationships;
2. Break cycles of suffering, alienation, abuse and dysfunction in the family;
3. Address parenting problems and painful family situations such as divorce, single parenthood, miscarriage, infertility, abortion, adoption/custody);
4. Deal positively with severe illness and death
5. Uncover reasons for physical and emotional suffering and take steps towards healing
6. Understand the "bigger picture" of any life situation
7. Create a solid foundation for taking a new, healthier direction in life

I went to the Family Constellation workshop with the idea of learning how to deal with my "challenge"—which is to say, to learn where it came from and perhaps how to get rid of it. I learned a great deal about myself with the aid of those representing members of my family and one person who represented "M.S." (No small task!)

Since undergoing this dynamic process, I have gone back as an "aid" to help others work through issues. And I must say that each return trip has deepened by understanding of how truly interconnected we all are on this planet, and also how healing at various levels can be facilitated by actively participating in "family constellation" exercises.

Dad ©

Dad was hard as nails mostly,
Not given to idle conversation.
Up by five not stopping for Sunday,
Just pounding, twisting,
Grooving, grinding, tuning,
Welding, shaping, fitting
Steel on steel
Serving
Impatient farmers....
Their mutual enemy,
Persistent, relentless time.
Demanding, scolding
Expecting, teaching:
The way it was in my learning;
So keen and schooled
In his ways
I could tear down and reassemble
A car when I was ten....
Expected of the first born son.

MA ©

Very private,
Ma was,
Soft as corn
In early summer,
Except when
She was busy
Which was
Always.

CHAPTER NINE
Human Guinea Pig

During the summer of 1997 I became a "guinea pig", as I called it, for a world wide clinical study of a new drug that addressed 'Progressive Multiple Sclerosis'. This was an outgrowth of my being very proactive, insofar as I had bugged research scientist and head M.S. doctor at the University of Washington Hospital in Seattle to do something to aid sufferers of multiple sclerosis. This culminated in my getting a call from the head of a one year UW clinical study in which I was asked to be among the 40 people world wide selected to participate. This study, I was told, would involve no use of a placebo. All forty participants would be given the "real McCoy" drug to self-administer three times daily.

It was just what I had asked for, the chance to be involved in seeking answers and a possible solution for this devastating "challenge" that bedevils the lives of so many folks all across the world. I signed on quickly and was promptly informed of what would take place plus possible side-effects.

The side-effects were not long in revealing themselves— nausea, headaches, fatigue and so on....uncomfortable for sure but not disabling for me, at least not yet. I could count on having an upset stomach each time I downed a set of tablets— —three times a day. I'd try to control the queasiness by eating Tums®—lots of them! I also had to wrestle with headaches and fatigue.

Having been active physically all my life, I felt that exercise might help the drugs and body work together. With this in mind, I put myself on an exercise program to increase my flexibility and balance. This consisted of "stretching" exercises to limber up my ole body, followed by some simple toning and strength routines such as sit-ups, push-ups and breathing exercises.

The drug and exercise combo did prove rewarding. After just 30 days, my walking and balance improved. However, my speech had slowed down somewhat. Sixty days into the program, my walking and stamina were still better than before I started the program. I even pushed myself to do things that I have not done for several years including—raking leaves, breaking up some sod for a garden, going on half mile hikes (up and down hills). I was a slow poke, but derived immense satisfaction from doing these simple tasks.

I hung in and took the drug and my "antidote" (Tums®) for the duration of the one year study. When the results were tallied up, I had gained little if anything from the drug. Actually, none of those involved got better save one woman, and no one involved could say for sure why. Maybe it was the drug, or just that she went into remission on her own. Of those of us in the majority—who did not get better—some (in fact) went backwards.

In spite of the nausea, headaches and etc., I feel it was worth the effort. If I did not try, I would always wonder, what if?

During September 1999 I took another shot at getting on the road to Wellness by participating in a study involving Procarin, a cream applied with a patch on one's skin. Basically, all I had to do was put on a patch with cream for 8 hours, remove it and put on a new one for the next 8 hours. Of the few other people I know of who used this drug, all appeared to have derived benefits to various degrees. I was not experiencing any improvements and had actually developed sores where I placed the patches; sores that spread to my arms, legs and lower back. Not surprisingly, I called it a day by later November and halted all use of Procarin.

By early 2000, I decided to return to Germany to visit with friends and to see Dr. Ledwoch at the Paracelsus Clinic in Langenhagen, just outside of Hanover. This trip included two weeks in Langenhangen, 5 days at the clinic doing their new Calcium EAP Intravenous drip method, with added vitamins. It took one and a half hours per day to complete a single IV drip infusion, then I was free to visit friends, sightsee or just rest.

After a 4 day trip to Normandy (France) to visit friends in Freneuse, I returned for the last round of IV drips and a final visit with Dr. Ledwoch before returning to the USA.

For me, the trip was worthwhile in its own right—just getting away and enjoying friends and sites in Europe. Upon my return home I continued the IV drip for two more weeks, than did injections every other day. I noted some small improvements, but nothing major.

During the remainder of 2000, all of 2001 and 2002 I experimented on myself using various herbal remedies and large doses of vitamins, along with exercise. There were no improvements, but no big losses either. It was hard to tell if it is helping or not, but the fact I was not losing ground made all this worthwhile to me.

During the early part of the new millennium I first heard tell of how stem cells could be surgically implanted or administered into the brains of MS patients, using tissue and cells harvested from aborted fetuses. This was something available and which I could do. I also learned that there were many risks, such as rejection or even developing a tumor somewhere down the road. The doctors at UW were quick to advise me against pursuing this sort of experimental treatment option.

Actually, I had no interest in this procedure mainly because of my belief that abortion represents the destruction of life, something I held sacred. Secondly, the term 'dangerous procedure' had been tossed out with reference to the stem cell implant experiment, something that caused additional anxiety. For some reason, I am nervous, big time nervous, when it comes to having some doc open up my skull and expose the "computer" that runs the entire show that is me. I was quick to rule out ever having this procedure done.

I was interested in stem cells even though my moral and personal objections ran high. The main thing that held my rapt attention was the fact that these cells could become pretty much any organ or tissue. It seemed, at the time, that there were many encouraging possibilities, but for me, not through brain surgery and definitely not using 'aborted fetuses'.

This went against everything that was taught during my youth, especially during my days under the tutelage of nuns both in public school and later on seminary. Of course, the very thought of having exposing the brain surgically added an element of *Frankensteinishness* to the whole venture.

Of course, I like most people had heard things about stem cells that didn't come from aborted babies; stem cells from bone marrow as well as stem cell-rich cord blood (umbilical cord stem cells). Bone marrow extraction and use left me a bit squeamish, but not cord blood stem cells. And while the experts seem to feel that cord blood stem cells were only good for treating blood borne diseases and conditions like anemia and leukemia, there were stories circulating concerning how some very primitive cord blood stem cells (designated CD34+) might help people with neurological and other challenges. As a lay person, I knew my limitations; which is to say, I could not lay claim to knowing what was truly possible, nor what downside (if any) might lay far down the road for those who use them. For me, the mere hope that these cord blood stem cells might bring improvement or even partial remission was enough to compel digging deeper in the subject.

Cord blood stem cells, I found out, are harvested from the placenta or cord that attached baby to mother. Ordinarily following childbirth the cord and the blood it contains are discarded. This fact alone actually changed the way I view stem cells. Initially I was against the use of "abortive fetus tissue" as a moral issue, but now in light of how natural sources previously discarded could be used to help others, I favor continued research and trials and the progress they will generate.

Of course, I quickly came to realize that opportunists weigh in with the rise of any new area of medicine or research such as stem cell science; scam artists who are fueled by greed and who seek to take people to the cleaners with faux treatments or "inferior versions." Thus it is important to we exercise due diligence in identifying the chaff and separating it out from the wheat.

One must also contend with the experimental nature of such things as cord blood stem cell use for non-blood born diseases and disorders. There are lots of unknowns, not to mention the fact that long term results that have accrued for analysis and publication in mainstream journals. Those who do such a treatment have no choice but to recognize and accept these limitations. Then too, like any treatment there are always going to be a certain percentage of people who simply respond poorly or not at all. Some drugs only consistently work well on 50% or less of users. This fact doesn't compel doctors to stop prescribing these drugs or people to stop trying them. Those who elect to have a cord blood stem cell treatment or anything experimental like it should make an informed decision, yes, meaning they know how things stack up. In many instances this places suffering people in the role of becoming "human guinea pigs" for the advancement of medicine—something I am intimately familiar with—whether within or outside of mainstream medicine and research.

With all this in mind, I had a cord blood stem cell treatment in Mexico at he hands of Dr. Fernando Ramirez, a Mexican trained MD who also had years of training in England (*University of London*'s prestigious Hospital for Sick Children) and the United States (*Wake Forest University, Brown University,* others), and was a highly qualified and experienced surgeon. Perhaps as important as credentials was the fact I instinctively trusted Dr. Ramirez.

But why get treated in Mexico?

First and foremost is the fact that the Food and Drug Administration (FDA) has not approved cord blood stem cells to treat anything outside of a narrow range of blood-related disorders. Research is going on, but so far it appears the only studies involving cord blood or cord blood stem cells for neurologic challenges are confined to lab animals. Many other countries such as South Korea are conducting clinical trials and administering or implanting umbilical cord stem cells into patients with such neurological issues as Lou Gehrig's disease (ALS) and certain spinal cord injuries. Some progressive countries are also sanctioning other types of stem cell use such as use of stem cells from the nose (olfactory ensheathing glial cells) to treat spinal cord injured people.

In addition, many independent impartial sources pointed to Dr. Ramirez as offering the most well thought out and safeguarded human umbilical cord stem cell program in the western hemisphere. This line of referrals ultimately led me to Dr. David Steenblock, a physician in California who operates the only clinic in North America (www.strokedoctor.com) that has developed procedures for prepping or priming patients' bodies to encourage the activity of infused or implanted stem cells. Encouraging too was the fact that Dr. Steenblock had founded a nonprofit research institute during 2002 (Steenblock Research Institute) whose staff of seven was busy collecting and analyzing data on the response of patients treated with cord blood stem cells by Ramirez.

Of course, I am not alone in going abroad for some kind of cell or stem cell therapy. A famous actor, injured in a fall, with spinal cord injury chose to have some kind of stem cell treatment done in Israel. Legions of people with Parkinson's, Cerebral Palsy, heart conditions and such have chosen clinics, hospitals and research centers in Mexico, Portugal, China and elsewhere for treatment.

JIM HAVERLOCK

Dragon drawing by Emily Laguzza

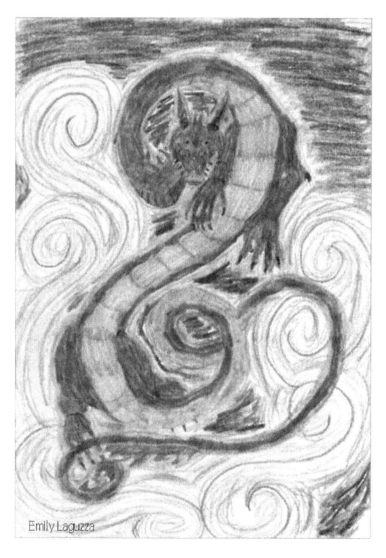

CHAPTER TEN
hUCSC Treatment

(umbilical cord blood stem cells)

The road to doing a human umbilical cord stem cell treatment was one surely paved with information, most of it provided me by Dr. Anthony G. Payne at Steenblock Research Institute (See *Forward* on page 00), as well as what I scoured from the internet. In order to make up my mind concerning whether to go to Mexico and receive a treatment, I wanted as many facts as possible before taking the "quick leap"! (Even though I am known for "jumping in feet first", thus my moniker—"flyin-blind")

After time spent researching (day and night over the next couple of weeks), I contacted Dr. Payne with a barrage of questions. He provided answers and I must say that I found him to be most honest and truthful as well as extremely helpful. After several more phone and "cyber" visits, it was determined the next step was a phone consultation with Dr. David Steenblock at the Brain Therapeutics Medical Center to learn if I might benefit from "prepping" for treatment in Mexico.

My consult with Dr. Steenblock went off fabulously. I came to find out that the Doctor was originally trained as a pathologist and was an expert at getting to the root cause of many chronic diseases. Then, too, he has a thirty year track record of innovation—like being among the first physicians in the world to use hyperbaric oxygen for acute stroke as part of a comprehensive neuro-rehab program.

Dr. Steenblock ordered blood tests and exams as well as a physical fitness test to determine if I would be a good candidate for a near term treatment with umbilical cord stem cells. He determined that everything was a "go" and I started doing the special "adaptgenic" prepping treatment regimen.

The following words are adapted from an MS web site I set up where I've posted my journey into the new frontier of human umbilical cord stem cell therapy (hUCSCT). It covers this time better then I could write it again.

It is happening—my treatment begins next week starting on Monday July 21st.

How do I feel about this? I feel like I'm on an emotional roller coaster. First off, I feel elated over the fact that this is really happening; that there is something "out there" that holds so much promise in terms of possibly improving my health and so many others in the same boat.

Second: I am excited to be a guinea pig again—though this time with a greater sense of impending success than was true doing any prior treatment.

Third: Nervous—yes, I would be foolish to feel absolutely no fear—for this is a trial, an experiment—but thankfully one that a few other people have done and shown marked improvement.

Fourth: Overwhelmed—that's a word I haven't used for a long time—but it fits. From finally making the appointment, to figuring out how to travel, finding a place to stay during this treatment, to gathering the necessary funds and getting them to the clinic for my prepping, wondering about what the future holds, how family will feel, how I share this with everyone...

Fifth: I started making video logs of myself—of how I am today to be followed by ones done on a regular basis following my treatment. This way I can visibly share this experience with others. And I did actually do a short segment today, and guess what? I was so surprised to see how I actually am, how I appear to others—which is to say, pretty darn scary!!! But it is me, and how I am...

Sixth: I will be leaving Washington state on Friday, driving by myself to California and—I must admit—I feel like an Astronaut, exploring new territory.

I am so excited——all went well. The drive down went well—took two and one half days to drive it, that's not too bad for me. Spent Sunday the 20th with my daughter and family in Carlsbad, then Monday morning (21st) reported in for my first adaptagenic treatment (This treatment involves lowering the oxygen level in one's tissues in a slow and systematic way, much like what would occur if one slowly ascended Mt. Everest. This is done because stem cells thrive in low oxygen environments). Following this I had a consultation with Dr. Steenblock (who does the post pre-treatment and post-treatment stateside—while Dr. Fernando Ramirez does the actual SCT itself in Mexico). At 3 PM I underwent another adaptagenic treatment, followed by a two hour session with Steenblock—a man I found so very thorough and so genuinely concerned about his patients. The same can be said of the entire staff at Brain Therapeutics Medical Clinic—all friendly, helpful and knowledgeable professional. I was especially impressed by Kevork Der Alexanian ("George"), a bioengineer and hyperbaric oxygen technician who administered many of my device treatments such as the adapatagenic one. He proved to be a truly wonderful chap, very compassionate and helpful and caring.

On Tuesday I had two more adaptagenic sessions, plus more blood work. Then on Wednesday 23rd, I underwent yet another adaptagenic treatment and then went to Mexico where Dr. Fernando Ramirez gingerly administered the stem cells—half subcutaneously just above my navel, the other half by intravenous drip method. It was a very easy session.

Following this, I was driven back to Brain Therapeutics Medical Clinic in Mission Viejo and had another adaptagenic treatment. This particular day wound down at 7:30 PM and I was back in my hotel room by 8PM—and slept until 8 AM the following morning!

The next day I had 2 more adaptagenic treatments plus an MRI of my brain and on Friday 2 final adaptagenic treatments.

I spent Saturday and Sunday with my daughter and family in Carlsbad (California), and was joined by another daughter from Phoenix who made a point of driving over to visit. On Monday I stopped at the clinic on my way home for a "booster" adaptagenic treatment. After this, I began the long drive home, arriving on Wednesday evening (30th).

Within the first three days following my hUCSC treatment I began noticing some positive changes. For example, after not being able to drink water for over two years—except in very tiny sips—I began drinking water normally. This was followed by a noticeable upsurge in my energy and clearer speech. YIP-PEE! To say I was happy for having taken this leap into the world of stem cell therapy is an understatement.

In the month that followed my treatment I noted additional little changes taking place in my body. Besides being able to drink water again, I was gripped by the conviction that life is brighter, my mind was sharper and clearer and I was really enjoying each day. My toes, which had been a problem for years—being curled up and looking for all the world like little hammers—straightened out. And I came to feel more stable on my feet, and was even able to walk about some without my support cane, and that felt wonderful.

Even my daily exercise routine became more enjoyable, no longer seeming like a "chore" as has been true in the past. I had purchased a "stair stepper" machine just prior to the treatment, and within a few weeks following my hUCSC infusion was doing 170 steps…which isn't bad for a guy with a challenge who is also an "old timer".

My co-worker, Pam Purtell (who has 3 children, 2 boys—Stephen and David—and 1 girl—Christina)—spends more time with me than almost anyone else. I asked her one day what she honestly saw in me that might have changed since my treatment. This is what she told me:

"I have noticed that your toes are uncurling and getting straight; your standing is much more stable and I don't worry about you falling over as in the past; you are walking some without supports; your skin looks healthier and not blotchy like before; you are more aware of your body; you have no more stomach problems—probably because of your diet; your outlook on life is brighter and you are even more positive and you are smiling more these days; and you are sleepy and tired now, but that is as the doctors told you would be for up to 6 weeks or so."

Those are her words—not mine.….and I won't tell you what else she said—it may damage my image, besides, why would you want to know how stubborn I can be? Oops!!!

Through all of this, Drs. Payne and Steenblock stayed in touch, almost daily. What a blessing it is working with these gentlemen and their staff. I'd be remiss if I didn't share a big "thanks" for them and all the world to read!

CHAPTER ELEVEN
DIARY OF A GUINEA PIG ON THE ROAD
TO WELLVILLE

One of the vital planks in my "self-repair-defeat despair" program is diet. But not the "3 squares" per day kind of diet that conforms to the official government food pyramid! Instead, I eat pretty much as people did before the advent of agriculture; before grains, cereals and cow's milk was introduced as dietary staples. According to many experts, especially anthropologists who study dietary patterns and adaptations across millions of years, we really are not all that suited to handle grains, cereals and milk (after weaning). There is, in fact, evidence that human health declined in many respects after these were introduced and spread among ancestral peoples.

This dietary approach is known as "The Paleolithic" or "Stone Age" diet, and is part-and-parcel of a regimen created by Steenblock Research Institute researchers as part of the body of technical support they furnish to the man who treated me with hUCSCs in Mexico, Dr. Fernando Ramirez. The diet itself removes common food allergens and compounds that tend to create inflammation, especially in folks like me with health challenges in the nervous system that actually generate inflammation.

The diet version for folks with neuro-inflammation like me is austere: No red meat, no colas, no sodas whatsoever, no alcohol, no grains, cereals or pastas, no dairy products, no coffee, no peanuts or cashews, nothing out of aluminum cans, and only certain kinds of fruit. However, one is a liberty to chow down on lots of vegetables such as cauliflower, cucumbers, celery, green, red & yellow peppers, spinach, dark green/red lettuce, summer squash, acorn & butternut squash, and a few kinds of beans (kidney, lima, green). Generally speaking, organic food is used as much as possible including free range chicken, free range eggs, free range turkey and small young trout, lake bass, salmon and catfish. Red grapes are good and so are blueberries. Foods with added sugar are held to a minimum. Nuts and seeds are a "no, no", because they rev up production of a chemical called nitric oxide in the Central Nervous System—which for MS patients is akin to throwing gas on a fire!

Yes, it is a fairly restricted diet, but I can tell you from experience that it is actually easy once you start, and you will feel better and more alive with each passing day. Literally! And this has proven true in the case of many other MS challenged patients who've gone on.

Thinking positive isn't part of the diet, but is part of my diet—my psychological diet. That is. I also exercise—as it is good for body, mind, spirit and soul—and make a habit of reaching out and helping others.

Following my first hUCSC treatment, I noticed that my dreams were taking on an interesting hue: Some of them were of me walking up a hill with a cane in the company of a friend. Suddenly I stop, pick up my cane, and say aloud "That's it, no more cane" and then I turn and take off at a brisk pace. Soon my friend is running up beside me, huffing and puffing and exclaiming "Slow down, I can't keep up with you!" The dream was in "living color" to boot, something rather rare prior to the stem cell therapy.

My skin, too, began taking on a healthy glow following my first hUCSC treatment. Not long after I got back from Mexico, I had lunch on a Friday with friends in the little town of Chelan, which is about 50 miles from Twisp. One of my dinner companions, Rob exclaimed that I "...look so Shiny". His partner added that my skin was more like "glowing".

Not unexpectedly, I had many folks asking me about the stem cell treatment and what I do on a doing basis to nudge the process onward. I found the easiest way to answer them was to share the nuts-and-bolts of a typical day. Here it is:

Most days for me kick off between 6am and 6:30am when I roll out of bed, get on the floor and start doing a specific exercise routine which lasts for about 30—40 minutes. This consists of some Alexander routines (see chapter 8), which is really all about getting one's mind and body working together. Then I do 30 sit-ups (up from the 8-10 that I did prior to hUCSCT), right elbow to left knee and then the other side, with increasing repetitions. This is followed by 30 push-ups, pulling my knees to my chest, one at a time, more stretches with the legs, some lower back exercises, then standing and bending forward to touch my toes (20 times). Then I stand and do deep breathing exercises by raising my arms and reaching for the sky, holding this position, than exhaling while crossing my arms in front of me so as to squeeze all the "bad air" out (I do this 30 times). I then do some isometric exercises like climbing an imaginary rope with both hands (20 times), then raise my arms above my head and link my fingers while pulling as hard as I can (20 times), followed by some bicep exercises, eye exercises, plus some "high stepping" on a stair stepper (230 to 280 steps per day, depending on how I am feeling).

Food:

The diet I follow is mostly raw vegetables, free range chicken or turkey, a little fruit, but no coffee, chocolate, sugar, grains, breads, dairy products, potatoes, tomatoes, nuts or seeds, nor processed foods and red meat. What at first glance sounds like a lackluster diet really isn't. The protein and complex carbohydrate choices are rich and diverse, and I find it a refreshing change from the S.A.D. (Standard American Diet). It pays dividends fairly quickly too: I trimmed up nicely over my first 3 months on it, losing about 20 needed pounds, and have been able to maintain this ever since. The nice thing is that I never feel like I am starving. Indeed, though I am eating less, I feel satisfied. But like most folks I am not above temptation. I ate one meal that did not fit into my diet and did not feel good for almost a full day.

Supplements and vitamins:

Sometimes I feel like a walking "vitamin pill box", but this is not something negative at all. The nutrients and such I take are meant to aid my body, and from what I can tell this is exactly what they are doing.

Morning:

I take 2 immune system benefiting capsules of the Tibetan herbal drug, Adaptrin on an empty stomach, then a couple hours later I have a small breakfast which normally consists of either some blueberries and and a 1/4 glass of blueberry or red grape juice to which I add 15 drops of "ginseng liquid". I then take 4 Calcium EAP tablets, one B12, one Folic Acid, one Cognicine (for memory), one high dose slug of vitamin C, one Curcumin C Complex (Anti-inflammatory), one GABA

Plus (Niacinamide), one A (10000 IU) & D (200 IU) capsule and since I am older and a man, I take one standardized Saw Palmetto softgel.

Noon/Lunch:

Lunches often consist of a salad blend containing spinach leaves or dark green luttuce, topped with chopped cucumber, radishes, green onions, summer squash, cauliflower, a small amount of broccoli, peppers (green/red/yellow) with some vinegar/oil dressing. I chase this Stone Age feast down with four more Calcium EAP tablets, one GABA Plus, one Cognicine, and one vitamin C.

Snacks:

My snacks would best be characterized as "Snack Lite": A few cups of green tea during the day and water, plus the odd bunch of red grapes.

Dinner:

I love home-made vegetable soups and so during autumn especially, I make a borscht soup with a rich mix of veggies, plus beets and red cabbage, seasonings, and a small portion of either chicken or turkey. Sometimes I will steam some veggies along with the chicken or turkey.

And on occasion I will bake some salmon or farm-raised catfish with a garlic/crushed walnut/olive oil topping. Nothing fried, of course. I finish this off with four Calcium EAP tablets and one Saw Palmetto softgel.

Evenings:

Prior to turning in at night I consume 6 prunes. However, on some nights I make and eat air-popped popcorn.

Sundays:

Sundays are "splurge day". I make an oven baked egg/veggie breakfast that consists of:

Summer squash, egg plant, red onions, red/green & yellow peppers, a leek, cauliflower, broccoli and spinach, all chopped fairly fine, some fresh garlic, a little ginger, cayenne pepper, dill weed, a small amount of feta cheese, some turkey bacon (cooked first and crumbled or chopped small), all of which is then placed in an olive oil sprayed baking dish. I then pour over this six farm fresh eggs, 1/2 cup rice milk (non dairy), 1/4 teaspoon of baking soda, and a dash of nutmeg. I cover the dish with tin foil and bake for 40 minutes at 350F, then remove the tinfoil and bake another 5 minutes. That's it, except for chowing down!

Gleamed from the Pages of my Personal Diary—November 2003—September 2005

Life is but a "moment" in the infinite expanse of time in the universe.

No matter if one lives a short life or a very long one, our tenure here truly is but a tick on the cosmic clock. What is important, at least to my way of thinking, is to get the most out of whatever time one has. I pull this off in many ways as these excerpts from my personal diary (Nov. 2003) illustrates. This entry was made only a short time after my first stem cell treatment.

Walking: I went to church on Sunday and as I walked from the car to the church I became aware of the fact that my toes were not dragging with every step. I paused, than started again for the church, but this time was focused on what my feet were doing. They were actually moving heel then toe, heel, toe, heel, toe...., than I noticed that the act of lifting my feet was now unencumbered. For someone who does not know the difficulty in moving two dead tree trunks when "walking", this may sound trivial. However, when your toes and feet have been wearing out the tops of the shoes for several years, this is major stuff!

Granted, I am not aiming for distance (yet), but to me these "small steps for one guy" is a much desired and welcomed improvement. Plus it is a sign these new stem cells are working overtime to affect some sort of overhaul on my aging vehicle (body). It's almost like taking a 1970 something car in for a "major" overhaul such that it will run for a few more years. And I want this vehicle (body) to "run" for quite a few more years!

I understand that life is short, of course, and that I have lived a good number of years already. Yet I feel that I have many more years left and it will be oh so nice to live them in a body that functions better than has been the case for the past ten years. Oh, yes I've both thoroughly enjoyed and made good use of these years, pruning and caring for my spiritual garden especially, which is all I get to take with me when I do leave this planet. But being around to enjoy another sunrise or sunset—well, that's something I want to do for a while longer yet.

My speech appears to be getting better, but it still varies day to day with the stress of work, and especially when I take a slight cold or experience nasal stuffiness (Something that happens all too often here in the North Cascade Mountains where the weather changes daily, especially in the fall). It can be in the 70's one day and in the 30's the next. This kind of roller coaster ride does tend to clog my nose and drag my speech down a tad.

Work? It amazes me how many hours I can now go

without being "fatigued" and wanting to crawl off and get horizontal. I am not like my adviser, Dr. Payne (Steenblock Research Institute) yet, who gets by on 4 hours of sleep each night and is never tired and always full of energy, but I feel that I'm doing better all things considered. And I'm now going from 6 AM until 11PM almost every day, which is pretty darn good.

Mid November:

During the past 10 days I have noticed slight changes. One of those is "more feeling" in the parts of my body that were "numb" to sensation. For example, I had a "pedicure" a few days ago and I could really feel whenever the manicurist cut the nail too short or applied intense pressure. This is something I would not have noticed in the past. Of course, the poor gal who did my toes was scared she was hurting me. We laughed and inwardly I felt good knowing the sensations were there and that I could actually feel pain. Indeed, it's amazing how good pain can make one feel!

Another change worthwhile came to light while I was having lunch with two acupuncturist friends, a husband and wife team. We had not seen each other for most of the summer and, after exchanging hugs, kisses and greetings, they both beamed as they noted that I "look so good, you actually look ten years younger." These were wonderful words to me—like water poured on scorched Earth!

I also am walking a bit more—without aids—around my house. This feels good. And I am still doing my exercise program, taking supplements and eating healthy. In fact, I had a short doctor visit on Tuesday morning, and per normal, they took my weight. I had shed 24 pounds since launching into this diet. What is even better is the fact that I feel so much better, am satisfied eating less, all the while the body is getting essential nutrition and is chugging along admirably. Yes, I miss the occasional glass of wine, and my favorite drink, coffee lattes. But when I get the urge, I just think of how much better I am and the urge leaves. I have been told I can have an occasional latte now, so I am waiting for a special occasion to do that. Perhaps Thanksgiving!!!!

Mid December 2003

Washington State has been in the grips of a flu epidemic. Many elderly and sick people have died. I, too, picked up the bug which took me down for most of the past 3 weeks. Down but not out! This was one nasty seasonal dragon and I am most happy to be feeling better now. My symptoms? Nausea, fatigue, soreness and aches all over my body, especially upper back area and chest. I also suffered from a complete loss of energy, such that I wanted to make like a cat and go find a corner to curl up in and hide from the world. And that is pretty much what I did.

One other thing is worth noting: Most MS patients in my position have compromised immune function. So when I got this virulent bug, I should have been down for the count. I wasn't. Was this good fortune, my natural constitution or a reflection of how my stem cell treatment might have in some way reved up or augmented my immune system? I believe the latter to be case.

There is one other thing worth setting down in writing: When I went in for pre-stem cell treatment exams, my Doctor told me he found a small nodule on my prostrate. He said this was something that I should have examined during the next 2-3 months. I did this—during this very month (November)—and to my relief he could find no sign of the nodule at all. This was,

I might add, the longest, most uncomfortable prostate exam I ever went through, but worth it in terms of the outcome and the peace of mind this engendered. I attribute this to changes brought about by my stem cell therapy.

Mid January 2004

Mid-January found me headed back to Mexico for a second stem cell treatment, secure in the knowledge that this treatment conforms to the best of medicine: It does no harm and either helps or does nothing.

For me, hUCSCT has been rewarding in so many ways, including the physical improvements noted of my first round. There are other ways it has benefited me too such as: All the new people that have been drawn into my life; increases in my knowledge of the nature and course of multiple sclerosis, as well as natural foods that can keep the body going and maybe even slow the disease's down; and, perhaps most important of all, the joy and privilege of helping others. I've also learned how important it is to never give up; to keep striving towards better health and independent living.

Post-Treatment

It is less than 3 weeks since the treatment, too early really to see much change. However, even so I have noticed a slight improvement in my finger dexterity; which is to say, that I find it easier to pick up smooth objects off counters or tables, such as the slippery Calcium EAP tablets I routinely take each day. Typing on my computer keyboard is also slightly easier and more on target.

At this time I am still not completely sure, but it appears my balance is improving. The reason I say this is almost comical: I caught myself in time to prevent suffering a nasty fall a few days ago, something I would not have been able to do previously. Indeed, for the past three years whenever I felt myself falling backwards, there was absolutely nothing I could do except hope that I would not knock myself out or otherwise hurt myself. On this particular occasion I became aware of the sensation, knew I was starting to go over backwards and was able to stop myself and get to an upright position quickly. This was a most welcome feeling—knowing I had thwarted a fall and almost certain injury.

My usual routines of exercising, cooking, cleaning, and working continue pretty much on target as before, with slight improvements in each. Pam, who works with me, Ron (a very good friend) and Sharon who works at one of the factories we buy from, have mentioned that my speech is again improving and getting stronger.

SMILE!—Mother Teresa said: "Every time you smile at someone, it is an act of love. A gift to that person, a beautiful thing."

March 2004

I had an adverse reaction to a new supplement added to my regimen. This put my life on hold for a time. Seems a combination of two of these caused a form of the blues to set in, such that my body, mind and emotions were down so low as to lend me to not care about much of anything. Indeed, I was well on my way to becoming a recluse. Once the reason for this "depression" was determined and my supplements and such were stopped for a time, my body, mind and spirit slowly returned to "normal", and with it my usual positive attitude.

I will give my ole body and mind a little more time to settle down properly and then pick up sharing my changes with the world. In the meantime, my speech has improved some and life is again looking bright and cheery. There is no one to blame for things like this happening, it is just part of the trial and error "experimentation" that is needed to figure out what works best for me. I went into this entire process knowing it is experimental, and by being a willing participant. And, I am still most happy that I have chosen this path and am thankful for the improvements seen thus far. I remain positive that more improvements are forthcoming.

Mid March 2004

Shaking off the depression caused by a combination of drugs last month has been a blessing indeed. Feeling good is so much better than that "blue funk" and life is indeed brighter. This helped me to better understand those who live with depression, or at least go through extended bouts wrestling this particular dragon. It helps me be more sympathetic by knowing that a chemical imbalance, whether induced by drugs in my case, or by a bad times or "bad genes" can make life miserable and affects one's thinking. Life continues to teach, inspire and humble me.

From the look of things my latest stem cells dose is working slowly this time, though there are some slight improvements as noted previously. None are as quick and noticeable as the first treatment, and I do fully realize that each stem cell recipient may have varying responses. So far, I have seen improvement in my ability to stand without support, as well as my balance and speech (Though admittedly both vary from day to day depending on the amount of stress I allow into my life). Overall, I am happy with the results I've seen to-date.

Yesterday I was up early and at work by 7:30 AM, on the telephone discussing business with others in various parts of the country; then at 8:30 a client stopped in for a short discussion, and at 9 AM I drove 40 miles to another small community to fill two new drug prescriptions. A friend decided he wanted to ride along and have breakfast. We got back after 1 PM and I returned to work where I hung in until 6. Then I prepared and ate my evening meal, did the dishes, cleaned the floor in the kitchen and bathroom, read a book (Gospel of Thomas) for two hours, then retired to the bedroom where I read some the newest issues of the National Geographic.

Most days I work 10 to 12 hours at the internet business I created, take care of my daily needs and chores, do some research and study on Multiple Sclerosis and spirituality. I also answer e-mails for other folks with MS. Along this line, one of my biggest thrills is when another person with MS whose done hUCSCT contacts me and fills me in on improvements she is having, or the spouse or significant other calls to express their happiness over his mate's improvement. The most awe-inspiring calls are from parents who are overjoyed at seeing improvements in a brain-damaged or otherwise challenged child.

Sometimes you take one on the chin—March through May 2005

Within an hour of taking the first dose of a new "trial drug", I found myself curled up fetus style, with what seemed like muscle cramps in every muscle of my body including my neck muscles! The pain was intense and I was shutting down to the point I could not talk at all, only lie there in tears. Pam, who works with me, came into the room and pretty much panicked at the sight, leaning over me while I whispered to call the doctor as to what to do—which she immediately did. He had me stop the drug right away.

The pain and fetus ball phase lasted for 4 hours, than my muscles relaxed. Being tired, sore and even grouchy, I asked

Pam to go home as I was headed to bed. My body went into contractions again at about 10 PM that night until 2 AM. There was nothing that I could but lay there in tears until it subsided. My body was weak and totally pooped out when the spasms at last dissipated and I at last fell into a sound asleep.

The next morning (Saturday), I slept in and did nothing the entire day except to entertain Ron, Pam and a next door neighbor who all came to check up on me. It is so good to have caring friends and neighbors and I know that I am blessed for it.

It turns out this new drug was a "scam" item that originated in another country. It took a few weeks for this to become known and during this time my body was recovering very slowly. Needless to say, my friends thought I was dying for sure, and were happy I did not. Me too!

As it turns out, this drug not only almost took my life, but put my M.S. into high gear. The autoimmune assault on my central nervous systems (CNS) was now (it seemed) taking off like a loaded down semi careening down a steep mountain!

Over the course of the next few months these ongoing attacks managed to pretty much reverse all of the improvements made by the stem cell treatments, plus pushed my body into a downward spiral.

My speech declined to the point I could no longer converse with customers on the phone and had to relinquish this pleasant aspect of my work to Pam and staff. It became so bad that every attempt to speak was done with great difficulty.

Gains I'd made previously in mobility were lost and in time I declined to the point that a power chair was needed and pretty much became "home" on a full time basis. My energy level also sagged, muscle spasms became more frequent and by the end of each day I was ready to hit the sack promptly.

During these miserable months, Dr. Payne and I conversed on an almost daily basis. He provided me with many ways to keep my body healthy and chugging along, including ideas on how to slow progression. Dr. Steenblock chimed in too and requested new tests to determine where this body was at. The plan was to get it prepped for yet another umbilical cord stem cell treatment.

Over a period of many months I had samples of blood and such taken and shipped off for testing, got results back along with a prescription for various dietary, supplement and other measures. Slowly but surely I came out of my nose dive and began climbing skyward. However, the loss of past improvements coupled with new losses were damn discouraging, to put it mildly.

By the end of August, 2005, it was at last determined that I was ready for the next round of treatments with September 13th being my "launch date". I purchased plane tickets, arrangements were made to have Dr. Ramirez in Mexico perform what would be my third hUCSC treatment, and I received word that my daughter and her family down in southern California would be happy to provide a place to stay (Thus giving me a wonderful opportunity to also spend time with some of my grandchildren).

On the sunny side of the valley again—August 2005 onward

Following my hUCSC treatment I began experiencing improvements. My speech has reached a point I am no longer afraid to talk to friends and I have begun to do more visiting. Also, when the phone rings at work and everyone else is busy, I answer it and, although I speak very slowly, find that customers understand me.

My energy levels are increasing, and my mind seems clearer

and sharp again which helps make work much more tolerable and enjoyable. New work-related ideas are again forming in my noggin and are being implemented. I have also begun getting out of the power chair and doing some walking. The walking is awkward, but for short distances it is done without canes, walls, furniture or any other type of aids.

All of these developments have placed my life on the sunny side of the valley and engendered hope for the future, not only for me, but for the many others who share my affliction and who have done or are considering doing hUCSCT. The future is looking bright for those who are "challenged", and the Dragon may well take a fall or two in the near future.

CHAPTER TWELVE
CHALLENGES—VALUES

Providence has hidden a charm in difficult undertakings, which is appreciated only by those who dare to grapple with them."

This saying, for me, is about as "right on" as one can get! When one accepts a challenge and then works through to a solution or victory or gain, then we are better able to savor the experience. It's easy to shrug off a challenge, to think that it's too big a risk or a waste of our time. But to take on a challenge, to grapple with it, can lead one to a place of discovery; of finding out just what we are capable of, and that is beautiful in its own right. My "Challenge" is a daily one—grappling with MS—a process that has opened up a world of insights and discoveries, plus many adventures. What about yours?

I believe that one of the most formidable challenges we all seem to be facing is a steady erosion of our basic values. There is today a lurking evil as insidious as the M.S. I wrestle with; a dark, malevolent dragon that devours all who cross its path: *Self-righteousness.* The tendency of folks to rationalize and justify just about anything they do; to excuse the most reprehensible conduct on the basis of contingency, pressing need, expedience, ego or selfishness.

Self-Righteousness

Doesn't just about everyone feel their particular spin on reality and beliefs justify their actions? This, to my mind, is the inherent danger in all self-righteousness: That anyone can become righteous in their own eyes, from the killer who justifies his violent rage, to ecclesiastical demagogues and political extremists of all colors and stripes.

By distorting or ignoring facts or logic or what is fair or just, it is possible to build a house of cards and then justify almost any act that rubs against all the noblest qualities and ideals of humanity. Indeed, have not all wars been started by men who were "righteous" in their estimation?

A CHOICE ..

Wouldn't it be nice if everyone would......

Choose to be easygoing, forgiving, compassionate and unconditionally loving towards all life in all its many forms and permutations without exception, including ourselves? To focus on unselfish service and the giving of love, consideration, and respect to all creatures?

To...avoid negativity and the pitfalls of worldliness and its insatiable appetite for material possessions and wanton pleasures? To forego rash judgments and harsh opinions, the vain quest for always being "right" or #1, and the trap of self-righteousness?

To.... seek to understand rather than to condemn? To venerate teachers of these basic principles and ignore those who teach or live contrarily? To apply these principles to one's self-view as well as to others? To trust in the love, mercy, infinite wisdom and compassion of Divinity which pierces all human error, limitation, and fragility? To place faith and trust in the love of God, which is all forgiving, and understand that condemnation and fear of judgment stem from human ego? Like the sun itself, does not the love of God shine equally on all of us? Should we not avoid negative depictions of God, especially those images and characterizations that are reflections of ourselves (That anthropomorphize God with human-like jealousy, anger, destructive fits, bias, vengeance-seeking, insecure, vulnerable, etc.)

Should we not substitute humility for vanity? (Vanities include: Holding opinions to be fact, judging others without just cause, and posturing). Let go of "I", "me", "mine" and use impersonal statements.

IF WE ARE ALL ONE ..

Then doesn't an action or thought that we have affect everything and everyone?

11th Commandment?

Most of us know something about the Ten Commandments championed in the Hebrew Scriptures, but how about an addendum? An 11th commandment? Jesus in the New Testament is reputed to have said: "Love one another as I have loved you."

Reading through the New Testament (which is comprised mostly of letters written after the death of Jesus) provides information regarding the life of this seemingly charismatic rabbi and how he cared for all the people in his orbit, whether infirm, blind, or afflicted with a dire disease such as leprosy. They tell of his love and compassion for them, and of his death at the hands of a powerful, corrupt empire.

Could I give my life for those I love? Or at least show compassion? How about just loving everyone? (And no, loving everyone because they are God's handiwork doesn't mean endorsing their wayward, sinful actions).

How about seeing God in all of creation? If we were to do that, then wouldn't it make it more difficult to harm other living creatures? Can you imagine a life with no more war?

Can you fancy how the world would be if we stood up to the challenges to our values; to the assaults on what we know to be right. And instead of compromising, what if we stood our ground? How many dragons that now send us reeling and threaten to utterly defeat us would we vanquish?

Friends ©

When did it begin?
Early,
Very early
I trusted Bo
As he trusted me
Laughter
Came easy
Then
He was loyal
Even when I was
Wrong
He understood
My pain
Where is he now,
I wonder?
I miss
My friend.

CHAPTER THIRTEEN
HOPES AND DREAMS

I nurture a lot of hopes and dreams, all of them empowered by the conviction that someday soon a cure will be found for many of the health "challenges" that are now incurable. This is an informed form of hope or faith, as new developments and discoveries are being made by scientists and others at an almost exponential pace. New technologies are being developed too, as well as new spins on the human brain, the thoughts and emotions it generates, and how it functions and interacts with the body in responding to all kinds of things we do, breath, eat and such.

It was new technology, in fact, that made it possible for scientists to zero in on and separate out specific stem cells in cord blood that tend to support neurological repair and such. One of these subtypes, designated CD34-/45+, is the one that was used to treat me most recently. And I understand that there are many more innovations in the works and that some of the brightest medical research scientists are working ever so quickly, with their main impediment being a need for restrictions, and of course, more money.

Something we can all do to help researchers do their jobs more efficiently is to pray, write letters to our leaders, and talk to everyone about increasing the funding of research.

Among the other hopes, dreams and observations (some admittedly controversial) I harbor and that may encourage some "healing of the soul" on the part of at least some kind readers:

Our knowledge of how this planet works and our role in caring for it needs to be expanded and its lessons acted on, not just given (our) intellectual assent. We need to acknowledge how we have disrupted the natural workings of this planet, how we have brought into being illness and resistant germs and such, and also how we have destroyed entire societies and parcels of geography out of greed, stupidity or a lurking desire to press everyone into our particular cultural or religious or political mold.

Surely all of us has some inkling as to how connected and inter-connected the ecology and societies of this world all are. Of how greed and lust have dominated us for far too long; of how we need to not only be *civil*-ized, but to live with compassion for one another, through helping , meet each other's needs, and through not trying to amass "extra things".

And to my way of thinking, it is now high time for all religions, Christianity, Islam, Buddhism, Baptists, Methodists, and all others, to soft pedal labels and the idea that theirs is the only "true religion," the only way to bliss on Earth and heaven afterwards. Religious folks also need to quit enabling cleric's control of others through fear and guilt, of their tendency to make their fellow parishioners and those outside their particular flock feel that the Almighty is pretty much a petty tyrant intent on stoking the flames of hell.

It is also incumbent on those of us who are Christian to truly follow what the rabbi from Nazareth (Jesus) taught and lived some 2000 years ago; a body of beliefs from which Christian principles were derived but not really heeded. We also need to pay more than lip service to the reality of who Jesus was and what he stood for: He was, after all, a Jew born into a Jewish family, who delivered sermons meant for his people alone, who wound up betrayed and then executed at the hands of corrupt Romans on a trumped up charge of treason.

And we (I speak again of Christians) desperately need to reform the reformer; by this I mean purge our houses of worship of picture depictions of Jesus with blonde hair, blues eyes, and fair skin. He was a Middle Eastern Jew, not a Swede or Norwegian!

It is my conviction too that humankind simply must stop launching wars in the name of God. The God I believe in, the God who set this amazing universe in motion, and this earth and everything on it and in it, needs nothing from us humans other then to live the life given us to the fullest and to honor the Creator in all we do.

I find myself asking—rather frequently—"If God created everything, and is everywhere, then why does this creator need (or needed) blood sacrifices from part of His creation with other parts of His creation?" Isn't that cult-ish? Isn't that like "Paganism" that is condemned by the major religions?

Why is it right for a particular religion to impose itself on others around the world, such as what is happening in Africa, and what took place here in the USA with respect to American Indians? Does might make right? Is God a champion of fear, torture and terrorism? I think not.

I believe that people are becoming aware of religious shortsightedness and arrogance, and are finding their way to genuine spirituality as opposed to living by manmade rules that were never intended by God or by Rabbi Jesus.

In my case, I was raised a Catholic, studied at a Catholic Seminary in order to become a Catholic priest and a "Missionary". It is only now, so many years later, that I have come to realize that most "conversions" down through the centuries were forced on people; that those who did not convert peacefully were greeted with torture and sometimes death. Church history is awash in such things as antisemitism, pograms, inquisitions, crusades and so called "holy wars". I also have come to realize how much of Catholicism and most other faith traditions are built on human generated rules and beliefs.

And what is holy about killing and destroying God's creation, I feel compelled to ask?

Perhaps it is time for us to "love" all creation without "judging" it or trying to squeeze everyone or everything into a single mold.

Let's face it, throughout history religion has been the number one cause of wars and human misery. Religious belief fuels most guilt—and this born of man-made rules and regulations imposed by often corrupt men who sought control over others. I personally believe it is time for us to open our eyes, hearts, and minds and not embrace everything spoon fed us by religious leaders. Maybe then we can stop inflicting wounds and begin healing the many ills that bedevil us all. *Maybe then we can begin slaying the real dragons instead of the ugly, horrid ones of our own creation!*

A passage from the prophet Micah (Bible) is one of the most simple and compact expressions of faith. In a few words Micah answers the question: "What does the Lord require of you?" His Answer:

> *To do justice,*
> *To love kindness,*
> *To walk humbly with your God.*

It is up to me—-
To Practice—-

Loving God,
Loving all of God's Creation
see God in Everything, everyone and everywhere.

EPILOGUE

My heartfelt wish for everyone:
May your life be lived to the fullest enjoying each day as if it were the only day you have left to live.

And for those fellow "challenged" people I pass along the words of Mother Teresa:

"God only gives us what we can handle. I just wish he didn't trust me so much."

May you find your "challenge", whatever it might be, a learning tool that encourages growth with joy, peace, love and compassion.

And always, always keep seeking......

SUGGESTED READING MATERIAL

Handbook on Umbilical Cord Stem Cell Therapy

Written by Dr. Anthony G. Payne, Ph.D.
Available free and online at—www.14ushop.com/wizard

**Human Umbilical Cord Stem Cell Therapy:
The Gift of Healing from Healthy Newborns**

by Drs. David A. Steenblock and Anthony G. Payne (Basic Health Publications, March 2006, $24.95 hardcover. Available on www.basichealthpub.com and www.amazon.com)

Sins of Scripture

by John Shelby Spong

God without Religion

By Sankara Saranam w/ foreword by Arun Gandhi

Power vs Force

By David R. Hawkins, M.D., Ph.D.

Of Water and the Spirit

By Malidoma Patrice Some

As I Lay Dying

By Richard John Neuhaus

Tuesdays with Morrie

By Mitch Albom

The Five People You Meet in Heaven

By Mitch Albom

Joshua

By Joseph F. Girzone

Rescuing the Bible from Fundamentalism

By John Shelby Spong—Bishop Episcopal Church

The Bible

(Read with an open mind and ask hard questions—there is much Wisdom and a wealth of good therein)

The Gospel of Mary Magdalen

By Jean-Yves Leloup

The Gospel of Thomas

Translation & Annotation by Stevan Davies
(NOTE: the above two Gospels were excluded from the Bible during the Council of Nicea)

Death of Death
Resurrection and Immortality in Jewish Thought

By Neil Gillman

Science and Religion Are They Compatible?

Edited by Paul Kurtz

23639